What People are Saying...

Eugenia Zukerman's new book, *Like Falling Through a Cloud*, is a masterpiece of inspiration, poetry, reflection, memories, and the heartbreak of discovering that one is having the early signs of dementia. Writing in the present tense, of past reflection, of moments of sheer delight—as well as moments of sheer horror—Eugenia has authored a must-read. I was going to say a must-read for those who suffer from moments of forgetfulness, but instead, I'm going to say it's a book for *everyone*. It transcends the particulars, becoming applicable to any situation you might find yourself in. That is the sign of a truly inspiring volume, a classic, and *Like Falling Through a Cloud* is a classic—for everyone.

The beautiful message that Ms. Zukerman has created in the astonishing, revealing, and inspiring book is that we all have life to live, dreams to dream, and human kindness to both give and receive. The author has always been an extraordinary talent, both musically and linguistically. In *Like Falling Through a Cloud*, she has written the unforgettable.

—**Judy Collins**, American singer and songwriter

In writing *Like Falling Through a Cloud*, Eugenia Zukerman gives her reader privileged access to her inner life, as she begins to understand and live with a recent medical diagnosis. As she describes the vast changes in her different states of mind in a series of poetic snapshots, Genie's artistic aura shines through with lightness, courage, and humor. In expressing the borders between fear, doubt, vulnerability, and love, Genie reminds us of the delicate balance between human fragility and resilience, and how poetry and music offer a balm when we are faced with psychic turbulence.

—**Yo-Yo Ma**, cellist

The most interesting writers of our time are creating hybrid literature that combines poetry, fiction, and autobiography. As we proceed in life, our way of perceiving the world changes, and few writers have the courage to depict this. Eugenia Zukerman—perhaps because she is a musician and a writer—has chronicled the music of the brain in an extraordinary way. *Like Falling Through a Cloud* is beautiful and riveting.

—**Erica Jong**, author of *Fear of Flying*

Bravery and inspiration come in many forms. In the face of dealing with her own challenges, Eugenia Zukerman has written a beautiful personal narrative that inspires bravery in the face of serious life changes.

—**Jaap van Zweden**, New York Philharmonic Music Director

Eugenia Zukerman has taken an experience and event that can be traumatic and brought light to it. Her poetic style of communicating the nature of her world in the face of this challenge is endearing. I believe anybody who is themselves or is having any family member experience some decline in memory will feel uplifted and informed by this highly special and unique work.

—**Herbert Pardes**, M.D., Executive Vice Chairman of the Board of Trustees of New York-Presbyterian Hospital

My sister, Eugenia (Genie to me), admirably always embraces the moment for whatever it brings. After recently receiving the diagnosis of cognitive decline, she was stunned but then took stock of how she felt and what it all means. A generous result is her beguiling prose poem, "Like Falling through a Cloud," in which she faces the mysteries of memory and self-discovery through change. In this short, yet revealing, sometimes funny, sometimes sad volume, she shares her experience and her candid self-perceptions. This compact volume has helped me as Genie's big sister (and a physician) understand what is going on far better than my empiric medical knowledge. This gem of a book should provide solace and insight for family and friends struggling to understand the complex issues of cognitive decline. More than that, it is a tale of bravery, strength, and healing.

—**Julie R. Ingelfinger**, M.D., Professor of Pediatrics, Harvard Medical School, and Senior Consultant in Pediatric Nephrology at Massachusetts General Hospital for Children at Massachusetts General Hospital in Boston

Heart-crushing poetry, eloquent typography, and stunning candor combine to make Eugenia Zukerman's voyage into the uncharted landscape of memory loss the most compelling book you will read this year. A brave journey beautifully told.

—**Letty Cottin Pogrebin**, a founding editor of *Ms.* magazine, and author of *Getting Over Getting Older*

I have known and loved Eugenia Zukerman my whole adult life. Of course, it was easy to fall for such a ravishing beauty, devastatingly diaphanous Diana that she is, but once hooked, more arrows felled me: a brilliant musician, to be sure, but also a brilliant and panoramically empowered mind and spirit, a captivating and pioneering tele-journalist and media advocate for the arts, an inspired and masterful writer, endlessly quick-witted and always an impassioned and aware citizen of the world.

It should come as no surprise, then, that when she discerned early signs of a potential and ever-unnamed usurper of mental acuity, her response would be to make us all traverse this frightening stage of her life by imbuing tragedy with transcendence in her memoir, *Like Falling Through A Cloud*. Eugenia's choice of telling this chilling tale of tenuous tendrils of cognition as aphorisms of light, fleeting and fleeing as dandelion seeds, is a true masterstroke. She paints the pages in serendipitous typographical free-verse, with the ease and urbanity of an Ogden Nash, with the nostalgia and romance of Nabokov, and ever with an endearing charm and more than occasional epiphany all her own. Never has a book made me want to laugh and cry in equal and empathetic measure.

—**Christopher O'Riley**, world-renowned pianist
and host of NPR's *From the Top*

Eugenia Zukerman bravely shares her personal journey and self-awareness as she battles with Alzheimer's and the anxiety that comes with it. She inspires with her strength and willingness to find joy and beauty in small and big things in life. Through music, love, family, and peace of nature, you feel her determination to appreciate every day and the will to move forward. She beautifully translates her frightening and inspiring experiences into poetry for the reader.

—**Yefim Bronfman**, pianist

If there is any writer who might awaken your love of poetry, it's Eugenia Zukerman. She plays with words in a way that makes you want to play with words in order to find humor, insight, and peace.

—**Alec Baldwin**, actor, writer, producer

EUGENIA ZUKERMAN

like falling through a cloud

A Lyrical Memoir of Coping with Forgetfulness, Confusion, and a Dreaded Diagnosis

EAST END PRESS
NEW YORK · BRIDGEHAMPTON

LIKE FALLING THROUGH A CLOUD

Published by
EAST END PRESS
Bridgehampton, NY

Library of Congress Control Number: 2019911526

ISBN 978-1-7324912-2-9
Ebook ISBN 978-1-7324912-3-6

FIRST EDITION

Book Design by Pauline Neuwirth, Neuwirth & Associates, Inc.
Jacket Design by Tim Green

Manufactured in the United States of America

10 9 8 7 6 5 4 3 2 1

To the end of Alzheimer's
and
to those who labor to find a cure

acknowledgments

I'm grateful to so many people who encouraged and helped me—
My great friends Oscar and Didi Schafer supplied their
encouragement
and support
Actress Mary Beth Peil led me to writer Denise Daily who then
introduced me to
publisher Pauline Neuwirth of East End Press and
publicist Emi Battaglia
that led to the publishing of this book

To people who worked on the book production, and distribution
I am so very grateful
To my daughter Natalia who helped with editing the layout and look
of the book I send thanks and a million kisses

And to those who cheered me on:
my daughter Arianna and her grand girls
music mentor Mary Lou Falcone
Investment banker/writer Beth Jacobs
Dr. Herb Pardes
and others
who pushed me through the clouds
to find the clarity I needed

to Claude Debussy with hopes to meet him on the other side

AND
to the love of my life, my husband, Richard Novik

like
falling
through
a cloud

like falling through a cloud

Sometimes

    when I wake up

it's dark

    where am I?

sometimes I know

    and sometimes

        I have no idea

so I let the night spirits wrap around me

    and they whisper to me

        Don't think. . . .

You will remember . . .

        I lie very still

        and

            then

suddenly

like falling through a cloud

      I know

      I

   AM

   HERE

forgetting

I told you
You asked me that already
Don't you remember?
What is wrong with you?
How many times do I have to tell you?
Why don't you listen?
Are you ok?
Don't you recall?
Are you losing it?
I think you're losing it
You need a doctor
Or something

YOU

   NEED

     SOME

      HELP !!!!

marbles

Maybe mine are lost
or maybe they're rolling around
in my head looking for a place to land
Or maybe not
my daughters tell me to get tested
tested for what I ask
even though I know for what
but it's for what I don't want to know
So I let the marbles roll around
in a swirl of distracting colors
because I don't want to listen to them
the daughters
because if I hear them
I will
be
very
afraid
and this mother cannot be that mother
not ever
never

words

they
    taunt me
tease me
    test me
when I fail to find them.
I know they're hiding
somewhere in the dark realm of my cerebellum,
floating around, mocking, sneering
shouting
Catch me! Remember me! Speak me!
Sometimes it's wise to wait . . .
wait for one word, or the kernel of the word
to explode like popcorn
and leap onto my tongue
bringing others with it
stringing a sentence together
for me to speak
and I say it, all the words
in the right order
spilling out of my mouth
and my brain asks me,
OK was that so fucking hard?

you don't have to tell me

I am no dope

I see how my family notes

my lapses and losses

of appropriate words

or a name

or the date

and

It makes me fretful

to be forgetful

so I try to hide it

but it's out there

the lapses and losses

which escalate

slowly

absurdly

inevitably

and I know

there is not a cure

for my fragile mind

but being no dope

I will try to find

the best way to cope

and I won't dance the woe is me

or bathe in a tub of self pity

I am not suited to it

I simply will not do it

I

will

find

a

way

my own way

which is the only

w

a

y

TO SURVIVE

taking stock, or so you know

I am a woman—72 years old

I have two wonderful daughters, a husband I adore, lovely grand
children

I'm lucky to still have a vibrant career in the arts

as

a flutist, writer, artistic director of major music series, television
journalist, educator   and internet entrepreneur

and

despite a little glitch with my memory

THIS IS THE HAPPIEST TIME OF MY LIFE

I won't joke about my Old Timer's Disease

nor will I call it early you-know-what

I am determined to remain centered

And in control and devoted to finding a way

my own way

to be able to say and to mean what I want to convey

and as long as I'm allowed to stay

I pledge to fight with all my might

to keep the darkness at bay

the consultation

I've agreed,
   grudgingly,
to have a consultation with an expert, someone highly respected in
the area of,
   what I am told is
           COGNITIVE IMPAIRMENT
   the which is what my
   family feels I am experiencing
(with the exception of my husband who does not
   agree that I am a candidate for this exploratory
      expedition, god bless him)
. . . but here I am and what I am feeling is fear and anger and
shame and
           HORROR
   But off I go with my younger daughter
   (the doc said it's best to have a family member with you)
         to the
      DEPARTMENT OF NEUROLOGY
   at a famous College of Physicians and Surgeons
(will I be drawn and quartered and put in a petri dish?)
     The facility is new and nice and looks clean
and when we enter the lobby, I am told to go to a particular desk
       where a pleasant woman
takes my papers and directs me and my daughter to the relevant floor
   —but nothing feels relevant to me here—
There are old people in the waiting room, most accompanied by a
nurse or a wife or husband. Some are in wheel chairs. Some are half
asleep or drooling or
        looking blank.

I may be 72 but I look younger, way younger, and I am still
cogent and capable and, if I may say, highly accomplished
and I want to turn and run out of this place right now,
but here we are, and when I am called in to see the doctor, my
daughter comes with me and there we are, both seated at a desk
across from the doctor who is the highly touted expert with whom I
will consult.
                           She smiles.
       I am surprised to like her right away.
             We begin to chat.
       What brings you here? I'm asked
And I answer: I seem to be having trouble recalling things—words
—names—places—and my family has noticed.
       My daughter nods agreement which is OK with me since I adore
her and suddenly I see why it's a good idea to have a family member
with me.
             Tell me about it, says the doctor
       I do have lapses, forgetfulness. I misplace things. I'm not as
organized as I used to be. It takes me longer to get things done. And
I sometimes feel confused.
                    How long has this been going on?
A couple of years, and yes I'll agree now there is more confusion
more forgetting
                                  and
my daughter, whom I adore, is beside me and she participates and
helps me with answers and time flies by casually until the doctor
asks a simple question:
       Is there a history of cognitive impairment in your family?
       My mother is one hundred and three, say I, and she's very
forgetful, but she's been sharp until now . . .
       More questions, more answers, and suddenly the doctor says
             We have to stop

and I look at my watch and it's been two hours.

I've given the doctor much information, which she says is helpful and she strongly suggests I come back for a

NEUROPSYCHOLOGICAL EVALUATION

and an

MRI

She says the evaluation will give her a good sense of where I am and it will help to decide what, if any therapy or treatment will be recommended

IF ANY?

How about NONE!

AND, she adds, the MRI will give us a look at your brain function

I want to say no thanks to it all, but

for some odd reason I feel

unburdened.

Somehow the terror that had me freaked feels somewhat tamed

but

I truly hope it will remain

U
N
N
A
M
E
D

my big sister the harvard doctor

She frequently talks with my daughters
and they've shared their concerns –
of course they have
because that's what family does
when one of its members is fumbling and
stumbling and bumbling.
I'm mad at them and sad at the same time
because I know it scares them
given our family history
which I had conveniently forgotten
until, after my consultation
when I called my big sister the doctor
    who reminded me that
SIX of our mother's siblings ALL developed cognitive impairment
quite early in
        onset
       AND DIED IN THEIR SEVENTIES!
  HOW IN THE HELL COULD I HAVE FORGOTTEN THAT?
    Because I wanted to
Because I must have had premonitions and
conveniently offloaded that information.
    Now I'm scared.
     Really scared
     And I tell my big sister :
I don't want to have an evaluation
    about my devaluation
    I don't need an MRI
      because why would I want to know
about my neuropsychological situation

when I can already tell it's all downhill from here
But she says to me adamantly
DO IT!

and
I know I'm sounding like a jerk
so
I stay silent for a beat
and then
grudgingly
finally
say

OK

evaluation

I will now be assessed, appraised, and evaluated by a person with a PhD who will determine how well my mind is functioning. I've been told that the testing will take two hours and I should try to be rested and feel well for my visit.

Oh sure!

My husband comes with me for support to this event at the famous College of Physicians and Surgeons at which I've already had my preliminary interview.

I pretend to be casual and unthreatened by the event until my husband is asked to leave the room so that the testing can proceed. I am suddenly no longer amused. I feel like a five year old being left off on the first day of school.

A lovely young woman with a PhD explains that she'll be asking questions and giving me some written tasks which are, for everyone, not easy, so I shouldn't worry about how many answers are right or wrong, but the test will help determine how I am functioning verbally, it will test my acuity, my this and my that and I am already anxious and I want to stand up and say sorry I can't do this, but I figure I can muddle through and it's not like I'm taking a final exam or trying to get into the college of my choice. Been there, done that

I voice my concerns:

This makes me very uncomfortable and nervous.

That's normal, I'm told.

I nod, feeling completely abnormal.

I'll be timing you with my stop watch. Some of it will be easy, she continues, and some of it will be quite challenging.

I think I'll like the easy part, I say

I'll be asking questions and I'd like you to answer as quickly as possible.

She smiles and I try to smile back.

OK says she. Name as many animals as you can that begin with the letter L as quickly as you can. And, GO! She clicks her stopwatch.

Lion, leopard, lizard, lamb, lemur, ladybug. . . . I hear my voice cracking and I manage to blurt out a few more L animals before I stumble and slow and stop and luckily she clicks off the stopwatch at the same time.

Good! she coos

It was not good and my heart is beating way too fast and when she quickly moves to the next question my head begins to spin.

I'm going to give you a word, she says, and I want you to rhyme it with another—for example, I'll say brother and you might answer . . .

Mother! I exclaim, like the eager student I've always been

Good—OK here we go, and she clicks the stopwatch, saying

Cricket

wicket I answer

horse–course

feather–weather

house–louse

collection–rejection

I'm kind of enjoying this back and forth stuff until I'm given a piece of paper and asked to draw a round clock face with a dot at the center and then, when given an actual time, to put numbers in the appropriate positions on said timepiece.

Easy! I think but I get all scrambled up and the flop sweat
breaks out on my lip and I announce, "I can't do this."

"You're doing it," she encourages. "You're anxious. It's ok."

"It's not ok!"

Can we proceed or do you need to stop?

Me? Stop? Me fail? No way. No, I'm OK, let's go on . . .

And go on we do and I fumble over almost everything

And once I'm done spending two hours with my interlocutor,
I am sweaty and exhausted and embarrassed and shaky.

AFTER:

My husband is escorted into the room and asks How'd you do?

Terrible. Horrible. I sucked.

She did very well, the tester tells him, on some things, and

she was less confident on others.

Then she turns to the less confident me—I'll be sending my
evaluation to your doctor and at your next meeting with her, she
will talk with you about the results.

"OK, then," she says, rising from her chair. "And now you'll go
down to the basement for your MRI."

"Yippee!" I crow, as a joke . . . which falls very flat.

But after what I experienced as a huge failure, I think I'll
actually enjoy lying in a cement tomb,

still as a corpse

while I'm bombarded with EXTREME NOISE

and magnetic imaging and radio frequency pulses

and indeed once I'm in my glamorous hospital gown

and strapped down onto a padded table

that slides into a tunnel as if into a crypt

and told to lie completely still

I feel more calm than I did taking a simple test to assess
the state of my obvious   d
                              y
                                  s
                            f
                       u
                  n
                       c
                          t
                             i
                                o
                                   n

the ride home

I'm sure you did better than you think.
I was a blithering idiot. It's like my brain blew a fuse.
Come on. You were told it was going to be difficult.
It was easy. A third grader would've done better.
You were nervous, that's all. You'll see, don't worry . . .
Don't worry? Are you kidding? I'm losing it. I'm skidding down
the slippery
    S
        L
           O
              P
                  E
Sweetheart, my husband says . . . and even though I adore
and admire this man I stop listening to him and feel my heart
pounding hard against my ribcage
    trying to
    break
    free
FREE of this horrible worry that my familial DNA is catching up
with me, and it's too
soon, I have so much to do, so much to experience . . . and I flash to
a vision of my future self unable to remember, unable to recognize
my children, or my
grand children, unable to speak or understand or . . .
    Sweets? My husband interrupts my silent soppy saga of
    imminent demise.
    What?
    How does dinner . . . and a roll in the hay sound?
    I laugh

Maybe, he says, we should skip dinner?
He touches my knee and I'm purring like a cat
    Yes, I whisper.
    Yes!

what's the point?

      I'm told
it will take several weeks before the results of my tests will come
through.
Several weeks without worry . . . before I know what I don't want to
know
          SO
   I plan to spend these days without thinking about IT
      because what's the point?
And I have a concert coming up so I have lots on my plate
     and I will just block IT out and
practice
     practice
       practice
Which is how you get to Carnegie Hall
    (and by the way, been there done that)
     meanwhile
I won't tell friends about IT
     because what's the point?
    It's dangerous—
   The word will get out—
    people will say:
     SHE'S LOSING IT
Even my good, solid, trustworthy pals will turn away
    or try to think of something nice to say
So I'll spend my time blowing my worries away,
   while I flute
     flute
      flute . . .

writing on the wind

Today I'm in a train
although some would say
   I am on a train
in and on and out I go and I am
going to the capital of our nation
by myself
with my own baggage
(literal and figurative)
to play my concert
at the Kennedy Center
which is no small gig
but although I no longer have nerves of steel
what I do have is my flute and
a lovely dress (one must look the part)
and a deep and devoted desire to
create luscious sounds and shapely phrases
by blowing across a golden mouthpiece
and there will be no words to jumble
or statements to stumble
    because
       sculpting sound with air
          is like writing on the wind

circles

Staying in DC at the Georgetown Inn
   Where I've stayed before
     Now newly renovated, lovely
      Near the Kennedy Center
And I unpack.
     I practice in my room
       hoping no one will knock angrily yelling
        STOP THAT NOISE!
       (no one ever has, but for sure one day someone will)
and then I take a walk through the crowded streets
    ambling aimlessly . . . .
      I window shop and have a cup of coffee
       and a chocolate chip cookie
but I get turned around and can't quite remember
    the way back
     but
    determined not to ask directions
 I
    continue
     to
      stroll
until I realize I've gone the wrong way
 but which is the right way
   and anyway what does it matter
it's a nice afternoon and I'll just keep going until I find the way
   back, but I'm tired and thirsty and I should probably hail a taxi
    I stop to get my bearings
   only to look up to see that I am
    standing

                   right
            across the street
            from
                   THE GEORGETOWN INN
so . . .
      I
            walk in and dig into my pockets for my key
                   but can't find it
I tell the woman at the front desk that I seem to have lost my key
and she asks
      what room are you in?
            AND
                   I
                   CAN'T REMEMBER
which makes me feel frantic
      I think it's on the second floor
            No problem, what's your name? I'll get you another card
THANKS I blurt but my heart is racing and my head is hurling
invectives at my
            completely
                   e m p t y
            b r a i n

confusion

        Clearly I am
Dis-
        oriented
Maybe it's fatigue
        or anxiety
        or both
so I decide to take a nap
        before the evening's rehearsal
and I fall into a twitchy worried state
        about forgetting my music
                losing my shoes
                        dropping my flute—
and what should have been restful was
        depressed-full
                and I wake up
                        with fear of failure
                on stage
                        and off—
        I try reminding myself that
I've played hundreds
        and hundreds of concerts

without being booed off the stage
        but,
                as I step into a cold shower
                        to snap out of it
                                I remember this:
                                THERE'S ALWAYS A FIRST TIME

get over yourself

Today there's a morning rehearsal

and tonight, it's show time!

I remind myself how lucky I am

to be able to make music with superb players

in front of an audience into whose ears I might

send sounds with my flute that can

move

or

delight

or

enhance

or

entrance

It's a chance

to paint with sound

to stir emotions

including my own

which have grown

morbid

with useless worries such as

    imminent demise

and an early

    unseemly

        DEATH

There's just one thing to do—

    stop feeling sorry for myself!

        Play my best!

  I will banish

    my darkest fears

        and

            Toot on

the ephemeral euphoria of applause

Relief
and a sense of accomplishment
especially
given the strange state I'm in
(and I don't mean Washington DC)

Backstage after the performance
kudos and kind words go a long way because
I'm no longer plumped with confidence
and although it wasn't my best ever
it also wasn't my worst yet . . .
I had a glitch or two
but perfection isn't the goal
now that I'm over my peak
but under my expiration date
now
I hope to walk off the stage knowing
I can still float an elegant phrase
and spin a tender melody
and tonight despite avid applause . . . truth is . . . I'm not sure I did

late that night, sleepless, i interview myself

How'd it go?
    It went
that doesn't sound very positive
    It wasn't a pig fuck but it wasn't great
So move on dot com
    Easy for you to say
You're nervous about next week
    You're right
And the test results won't be as negative as you suspect
    Oh yeah? They'll be worse than I thought
Worrying won't get you anywhere
    I can't help it
You can. You must. Think pleasant thoughts. Try meditating
    I forgot my Mantra
Make up another
    I donta wanna chakra
Funny
    Funny or die . . . I'd rather die funny than die sad
Somehow I don't think you get to choose
    That's really helpful.
Over and out!

interlude

Sixth grade . . .
members of the local orchestra
come to my school
to demonstrate their instruments
I hear the flute
    and
I am **enchanted**
b e w i t c h e d
mesmerized
    and
        I run home and tell my parents
I HAVE TO LEARN TO PLAY THE FLUTE PLEASE CAN I???????
and in those days long ago at public schools in America there were
instruments kids could borrow and there were music teachers who
loved to teach how to play them and at the age of ten I started to
take lessons and it made me happy and hopeful and blowing across
the mouthpiece to produce sounds was miraculous and delightful
and difficult but I wanted to do it, I did it, I played and played and
OK some days I hated it because it was hard but I had to practice
because that was part of the deal with my parents who were very
musical themselves and they encouraged me and helped me and
the first time I ever played on a stage was with my dad at my school
and it was pretty thrilling and I remember it was a piece by Gabriel
Fauré who was dead and very famous and I was scared but I did it
and I didn't mess up and that felt so good so I just went on taking
lessons and trying to play better and the flute started to feel like a
friend and when I would get home from school I was never lonely
because I could go to my room and play with my close friend which
might sound strange but that was how it was and it became more

than a friendship it became a love a deep and constant love and that's the way it still is OK most of the time but not always because getting old makes playing it harder so when I go onto a stage now I worry about messing up and especially now that I might be losing my cognitive function what I'm hoping is that my brain will remember where my fingers go and that I will be able to take a deep breath and exhale and send sweet sounds into the air because if I can't do that anymore . . . who

will

i

be?

back

I've returned to the city
 where everyone is busy
  and scurrying
   and worrying
and it's late summer
 subways are crowded and hot
  folks are sweating a lot
and the trains are
 always late
and some man gets up
 to offer me his seat
  which is sweet
   if somehow insulting
here's my stop
 I'm attempting to exit
I push my way out
 doors close behind
  but when I look up at a sign . . .
   this stop
    is
     not
      mine
   And worse
I'm totally turned around and can't figure out
 do I need to go back uptown
or change to the downtown track and how do
 I do that
  FIGURE IT OUT, BIRDBRAIN
   I wander around the station

looking for an exit, any exit
JUST GET ME OUT OF HERE
there!
stairs!
I stagger up
until I'm out
above ground
Out of breath
having arrived
survived
A walk home will be good
I need to get my bearings
but I won't be sharing
the story of my panic or pretty soon
I'll be forced to wear
a lovely bracelet
inscribed:
MEMORY IMPAIRED

at home

I live in two places
about which I'm of two minds
                    one:
 I'm lucky to live in two places
                    two:
I yearn to consolidate
                    because
my husband lives and works upstate
                    while
I live upstate but also down in the Big Apple
and although it's a privilege to have two beds
          on which to lay my head
I wish
          with increased concern
                    to stay put
                 to shelter in place
Instead of shuttling back and forth
     from south to north
and back again
     which
involves the high art of schlepping—
     flutes/clothes/shoes/books/music
          back and forth from abode to abode
forgetting what's where
     needing this when it's there
          I'm spoiled to care
     but I fear
          it might be part of the muddle
into which

I find
          myself
progressively
     slip-sliding
          d

               o

                    w

                         n

test results

A hotter than hot day
I take the steamy subway uptown
to the hospital
I'm early
which is one of my many failings
since it makes me waste time wandering around
waiting waiting waiting
which I've been doing for way too long
but here comes my daughter who sweetly offered to accompany me
to the gallows
and we
check in to the the Division of Neuropsychology
again
Wait wait wait
feeling scared as a fly as the swatter hovers overhead

And how are you? I'm asked when the doctor enters
Just ducky I almost say but answer I'm fine
Good. Good. And the test results are interesting
Oops, I think. Interesting does not mean good.

I hear papers rustling from which the doctor begins reading the
verdict:

Your premorbid intellectual functioning is estimated in the high
average to superior range, she begins, based on performance on a
word reading test and educational/occupational achievement.
Phew, I'm thinking. I passed.
But, she continues, basic auditory attention was low end of average.

LOW END OF AVERAGE? WHAAAT????? ME??????
　　　　　then
　　　　GOOD NEWS:
In contrast, tests of basic psychomotor processing speed were
measured in the
　　　　　superior range
　　and so it continued to go: up and down, good/bad
I hear results of my verbal memory my nonverbal memory my
language functioning my visiospatial functioning and emotional
functioning
　　AND I'M NOT FEELING FUNCTIONAL AT ALL
　　　　especially
when I'm told that "a salient finding of the examination was the
patient's profound anxiety regarding her cognitive changes . . ."
　　I TUNE HER OUT UNTIL I HEAR THE COUP DE GRÂCE:
"In the context of preserved functional abilities, her clinical
presentation is most consistent with a diagnosis of amnestic mild
cognitive impairment. In light of severe memory impairments
observed in the context of her family history, continued monitoring
is warranted to rule out a cortical neurodegenerative
　　　　process."
　　The doctor's mouth keeps moving but I am having trouble
following.
　　　　I hear salient phrases:
　　"Basic auditory attention was low end of average . . ."
　　　　LOW END?? MOI???
　　　　and
　　"your self-critical approach on testing..."
　　Well I flunked, didn't I? I'll never be able to remember
anything!
　　　　"That's what we call a possible maladaptive belief."
　　　　Meaning?

"Meaning of course you will be able to remember. But right now anxiety is likely exacerbating any existing weaknesses you might have which is making you feel that way. But," she quickly adds ". . . there is a therapy you should consider that can be very helpful . . ."

Great, I think. And what might that be?

Will I be bound and gagged?

Given shock treatment?

Will I be made to walk across hot coals?

"Cognitive Behavioral Therapy. It's a well-known treatment for anxiety and you ought to look into it. I think it could be really helpful—"

So now I need a shrink? I'm not keen on sitting in a chair and complaining about my childhood or dissing my parents or discussing one of my two past husbands. Been there done that.

"This treatment is quite different from talk therapy," the doc continues:

"It focuses on developing coping strategies that can help you solve problems and change unhelpful patterns in your emotional attitude and behavior."

Silence

"Mom?" my daughter prods. "That treatment sounds like a good idea."

"Sure," I say but going to yet another doctor? I'd rather stick pins in my eyes.

"I'll give you some recommended names . . . I suggest you give it a try, and we should re-evaluate in twelve to twenty-four months . . . ."

OR NEVER, I'm thinking as my daughter and I walk out the door.

Mom that's really good news!

What is?

The doctor says she doesn't need to see you for 12 to 24 months
—that means it's mild . . .
    What is? I ask, straight faced
she looks at me, worried
    until I Laugh
and hugging me
        my daughter
                        laughs too

reprieve

12 to 24 months!
I'm off the hook!
I feel absolved
forgiven for my forgetting
or so it seems
at least for the moment
I can roam free
from self blame and guilt
and get myself some help
some strategies
some daily schemes
to remember things
like my dreams
     BUT
how will I remember
what to remember if I can't
   remember
     what's forgotten
       or never known
and just the thought of that conundrum
     feels impossible to solve and makes my spirits devolve

task to self

Today I've promised myself not to fret
no worries, be happy
there's pleasure ahead
satisfaction, delights
cheery days, joyful nights
I need some strategies
some tactical schemes
and streams of thoughts that are
positive
productive
and helpful in
remembering
like a melody that repeats in my head
      SO
I'll give myself a task—
    to remember
  what I dream tonight
    and
be able to recall it
in the early day's light

morning baroque

I wake up not knowing

    where I've been or where I'm going

So I lie very still

and soon it comes to me—

my dream

A brown rabbit hops
harpsichord tracks
into my dazzled morning eye
where the rubbed vision
of night fades
obligati out
to focus on whiskers
twitching like plucked strings
and the gloved paws are poised
for the next chord.
The rabbit waits
   tips an ear
toward accompanying trees
and
     cadenzas
            off

dream catcher

Caught it! Remembered it!
Not perfectly
but perfection isn't the goal
If I can pull up my dreams
in the morning
I can pull up other things
like words and names that elude
Instead of what-cha-ma-call-it
I will remember what to call it
and not just dreams
but places and people
and where I left this
and where I lost that...
I'm jazzed, on a roll
feeling some control
instead of beating myself up
when I can't find a word
I'll let it slowly emerge
        like the call
            of a distant
                    bird

upstate

My husband laughs that I call it a farm
        but
   compared to my apartment
     in the Apple
    this place is large and luscious
with acres of hills and trees
    and a stream
and two barns and a big old farm house
  and bushes and brambles and animals
    domesticated and wild
and coyotes serenade us at night
 and a gorgeous red fox comes
down the hill to drink from the pond
and rabbits and chipmunks abound
and there's the garden my husband adores
he who fixes fences and feeds the horses
  and takes care of it all
    he who is the love of my life
I who adore being his wife
   so every day I pray
     my brain won't shatter
spilling all its gray matter

fluting on the farm

Just for the fun of it
    for the feel of it
        at 6 in the morning as the sun comes up
and my husband leaves for work
    and I'm not in my apartment in New York
so I will not wake a soul
    and the two dogs and the feral cat and
  the two horses
are already up to their outdoor tricks
    I open the window and play
    for them
  and for the trees
    for the flowers and the blue blue sky
for the squirrels and the bugs and the bluejays
    I play for the clouds
    I make up tales and stories with tones and tunes
and there are no words
  just a sarabande for the cat
a scherzo for the dogs
    and for the equines—a jolly jig for jumping

alone

I'm mostly home alone Upstate
    which is a state I don't hate
there's much work to be done –
    most of it fun
to flute, to write, and I have two music series
    of which I'm in charge
    as the Artistic Director
    and that takes a large
        chunk of time
inviting players, making programs, keeping dates straight
    talking to managers
  but I juggle it all and it's been great
    until
        NOW
    when I'm fretful about being forgetful
I misplace papers, I confuse names
there are two boards of directors to please
  and meetings to take
    and lately it's all a great big JUMBLE in my head
  but I tell no one that I fear I'm S L O W L Y
                  coming   undone

late august in new york

August—not just a month
but a word with weight
meaning
noble or grand
or so I understand
but in 2017 in New York City
it's more dis-gust than au-gust
it's a month of heat and horns honking
and bikes going the wrong way
and temperatures and tempers flaring
    I've come down from Upstate
because dreams remembered are one thing
but I find I'm forgetting names
  and numbers
    and tasks
like leaving a room to get something I need
and not remembering what it was I went to find
so on my own I've decided
to seek the expertise I've derided
and despite enormous doubt
maybe it can help me out

the therapist

It's hot in her office
and I suddenly don't want to be
    here
but I've made the appointment
and she's highly recommended
    by my doctor at the
famous College of Physicians and Surgeons
    so I'll give it a try
though I want to flee
and when she asks why I'm here
I say I understand you might help me with strategies to deal with
diminishing brain function heightened fears and a growing sense of
                            DOOM
    at which she smiles and says
I've read your doctor's evaluation—
    amnestic mild cognitive impairment
  with a self-critical approach and profound anxiety about
    your cognitive changes
SO, she suggests, let's see if your anxiety and your self-critical
approach
is exacerbating your existing weaknesses
    and I'm thinking LET'S NOT!
but now she's asking me to talk about my family
and I'm about to say NO THANKS when
she says I can be as brief as I'd like
and I want to say I have to leave right now
when what spills out of my mouth is a spontaneous
babble about the good and the bad of
a childhood with brilliant gifted parents who were hard to know

hard to please and always on edge because why wouldn't they be when my father had been President of Young Communists in college and Senator McCarthy was on his case and our house was bugged and my mother was always sad and there were secrets and lies everywhere and the polio epidemic to worry about and dangers galore and I was always on heightened alert and nothing I did seemed ever to be good enough despite fine grades and talent for writing and music and early admission to the college of my choice and success after and . . . and . . . and

    WE HAVE TO STOP NOW

says the therapist, adding, but I'm glad you gave me a picture of the young you, and it seems you grew up in a household where there was a degree of danger and dread and perhaps that's where your anxiety began to take root. Would you like to come again to talk some more?

    YES I blurt, thinking it couldn't hurt
        in fact I walked out of her office seeming oddly
            unburdened and alert

thoughts after the shrink

I've been a scaredy cat all my life
frightened by many things
like the car wash
horses
the bear hiding in the woods
ticks
tricks
losing my keys
or my Senior Citizen subway pass
sitting down without passing gas
sleeping alone
fucking up onstage
hitting a deer
It's gotten worse as I grow older
I would have thought I'd be bolder
but I've been feeling fraught and frail
and on a trail
that leads to nowhere
BUT NOW HERE I AM
walking down the street with a spring in my step
and I don't even mind the schlepp
back downtown
I'm
feeling lighter
the day seems brighter
talking was easy
I didn't feel queasy
about telling my tale
it wasn't a pass/fail

experience
    and I was surprised at the things
 I recalled
having not thought at all
I'd be able to dip into the deep
    past
the time went by fast
and now as I stride down the street
    I feel
little tinglings
    of something
        kind
       of
            like . . .
                could it be . . .
                HOPE?

determination

After my session
my takeaway is this lesson:
I've got to get me some grit
I hereby resolve to evolve to a stronger
state of mind and purpose
enough
whining and worrying and wondering
about losing my mind and ending up
wandering around town
blabbering to myself
barefoot in a ballgown
with my hand out for someone's kind quarter
the next step is to step up
and find ways to bolster my mind
and give me the guts to stop thinking
the red light is blinking
I may be in decline
but I'm not dying on the vine
not yet, I say,
not until they take me
away

september splendor

I walk up the hill
behind the barns
    where
The leaves are turning
from green to gold
awesome orange
the boldest bronze
  rusty red
and mauve
leaves flutter in the
autumn light
    like little flags
they shiver in the breeze
     fluttering as they please
       before they
    drop
        at my feet
like a confusion of colored confetti
        and I
     dazed by this beauty
       strangely
         begin to cry

hats off to hopkins (and his poem)

Now I get it, Margaret
why you're grieving
over goldengrove unleaving—
you with your fresh thoughts
me with my sad thoughts
but I weep and know why—
    indeed
It is the blight man (and woman) was born for . . . .
it is me I mourn for—
standing here in the woods
watching the leaves drift down
down
  down
    I grieve for
nature's beauty lost
    and
being tossed
    by the turbulence of time
and myself made sad
    by lamenting
my impending dementing

nocturne to overturn sadness

You rose from the depths of our sleep
and spread like a wave
your flesh on mine which woke
in my dream another dream:
Mountains and wildflowers
air cool as a drink
a thicket, leaves folded down,
a deer appears
He takes me on his back
I hold his smooth fantastic antlers
he leaps through the leaves
up slopes
down
slowed half-speed under the liquid sky
wildflowers, green, then blur of color,
kiss of wind
down slopes
up to the top
beyond—the long fall down
I woke and felt your breath against my cheek, up down,
    the heave of your chest
        like a deer just run

remembering to remember

I'm up first
his sleeping body relaxed beside mine
a slight smile on his lips
as if listening to someone's quips
and it comes to me so easily—
the deer
antlers
colors
wind
up and down and up and down
s
l
o
p
e
s
The sky a bright blue
like his eyes
that open just now
he smiles and I smile
because it seems
lying beside me, antlers removed, is the deer in my dream

love conquers all, maybe

Crazy about the man
I love him more than I
possibly
can
express—
more than today
and less
than tomorrow
as they say
and for 10 years
he's been the light of my life
no fighting no strife
just joy in the morning
    loving at night
but if incompetence grows near
I will make it clear
I will not saddle him
or rattle him
with the burden
       of a DEMENTED ME

getting over myself

I read the papers and worry
I hear the news and want to scurry
the earth is in a mess
and I confess
I think world war three is on its way
there's little one can say
to save the day
so what to do?
have good intentions
help out
pay attention
facilitate prevention
It's not a good time
to be in cognitive decline
but I want a chance to stand up
to the challenge of demise
look it in the eyes
and take it by surprise

close call

In my car
   check the rear view mirror
coast is clear
   turn the wheel
     pull away from the curb
nearly clipping a passing car
   he blasts his horn at me
     Phew!
    calamity free
yet the near miss frightens me
shaken I drive on
but how could I not have seen
     that car???
    What's wrong with me?
   am I crossing the line
between functional
and out of control
   as a driver I failed
    I could have ended up jailed
but I didn't
    which means I have to stay alert and aware
           or I won't be allowed to go anywhere

thoughts about a near miss

what's with me
one minute I'm on it, I'm in it
  I'm sharp as a whip
    I'm quick with a quip
I can charm and disarm
   then suddenly
I'm non compos mentis
  a killer in a car
I'm jangled and shaky
 feeling weak and ache-y
I'm back home
 it's a
Sunny morning
 chill in the air
   frost on the lawns
husband's gone to work
  dogs are out
    horses in the field
cat on the prowl
I've got a day
  to work
     play my flute
talk to friends
   make amends
for all the odds and ends
I've left undone
but I have a thirst
for Java first
grind the beans

pour the water
and wait
and wait
and wonder what's with
this damn machine
does it need to be cleaned
it's at least five years old
why isn't it perking
is there a glitch lurking
and suddenly I realize
for coffee to perk
one must
  first
turn the
  damn machine
    ON

back in new york

On the couch
　　but it's actually a chair
where I sit just opposite
　　the therapist
who asks me how I'm feeling today
　　I'm OK I say
except I'm forgetting to turn things
　　on and off
which worries me
not to mention I nearly
bashed my car into another
and I can't find things I'm looking for
or I forget what I forgot I was
　　looking for
and it makes me feel
stupid and inadequate
so I don't feel fine or fit
　　not the slightest bit
and I have concerts to play
things to do
meetings to take
for which I fake
that I know what I'm doing . . .
　　WHOA! says she
it's ok to be
　　the imperfect you
because you're able to see
　　your failings
but to beat yourself up

is not the key
   to taming anxiety
it's clear to me
that you need some strategies
   to stem the tide
that makes you slide
   into that
dark place of self reproach
    yoga might be good
or you could
      meditate
but it's getting late
   and we have to stop...
    SO
when would you like to come again?

and now i am suddenly seventy-three

Birthdays happen so fast
the icing on the cake doesn't last
long enough to remember how it tastes
and wrappings on presents go to waste
and despite dinner with friends
the evening somehow ends
on a bittersweet note as we age
but to rage rage rage
at the dying of the light
is a plight I plan to fight
so while losing my mind
I pledge to buck up and find
   ways to enjoy
       a new day
           every day
              in every way
til I'm certain
     it's curtains

getting it together

I've made a date
with my
banker
because I hanker
to know where things stand
when it comes to what I'll hand
to my next of kin
so I should begin
to keep track of stuff
to see if there is enough
to pass around
when I'm under the ground
I'm not being dramatic
but I can no longer be static
about what lies ahead
when I'm dead
which oddly I do not dread
         instead
I want to avoid leaving a mess
for the family to assess
I'd like them to say
she left it this way
to keep trouble at bay
and to avoid a fray
I don't expect to croak
at midnight's stroke
but I don't want to be
one hundred and three
which my mother's achieved

I will stick with the plan
I've made with my man—
when the time seems right
we will have the delight
of donning deer suits
on the first day of hunting
and we'll go out in the fields
and wait
        to meet our fates—
  only I hope
   the hunters know how to
shoot
        s
t
     r a
i
   g
h
     t

in order to promote tranquility and certainty

WHEREAS

The parties were married to one another in a civil ceremony

WHEREAS

as a result of their marriage the Parties wish by this agreement to
define their rights and interests in one another's property; and

WHEREAS

each of the Parties has been informed of his/her rights and
privileges in and to the property of the other under the laws . . .
and each understands that under law their marriage confers specific
rights upon each of them; and

WHEREAS

in order to promote tranquility and certainty . . . the Parties desire to
define and limit by the Agreement the interests, rights and claims
which accrue to each of them in the property of the other by reason
of their marriage to each other; and...

WHEREAS

If the parties are wearing their respective deer suits and each has
donned their

respective antlers, then each understands that the rights and claims
of the other

will be null and void if he or she should be the receiver of the first
bullet; and

WHEREAS

as a result of being the first receiver it will not matter diddly squat
who gets what
but let it be noted
that the certainty of tranquility will have been perfectly promoted.

the antidote to death

There are two grand babies now
and I still marvel at how
they arrived from the balloon
of their mother's womb
these gorgeous creatures from the blue lagoon
all parts attached and in tune
from the tips of their noses
to their wiggling toes and is
anything more astonishing than
meeting the child of your own child
and watching these tiny ones grow
and crawl and walk and talk
and the delicious hugs they bestow
upon the mother of their mother
for no reason other
than something in the DNA
that makes them feel that way
and one plus one makes two
little girls whose hugs and snuggles
erase all sense of struggles
these two little sprites
are my greatest delights.

so why do i worry so much about them?

The littles.
When my two girls were tiny
I didn't hover and smother
the way I do now
when I see how
my grands leap in the air
without apprehension or care
or kick a soccer ball
with all their might
which makes me fight
the urge to rush onto the field
and shout Stop! You must yield!
My stomach's in knots
when one of them trots
out the door and into the world
leaving me curled
into lots of hurled
self doubt.
Cut it out
Say I to me
And yet, and still, and always, I worry worry worry worry . . .

anxiety is inconvenient

I try to be lenient
on myself when I'm in a twist
about this
and that
I should make a list
about ways to avoid
self flagellation
and constant agitation
I should be able to grapple
with life in the Apple
and existence Upstate
it would be great
if I could just relax
instead of bracing for attacks
and worrying about cracks
in my brain—which is a pain
Maybe what the shrink says is right—
I need a variety of strategies
to fend off my endless anxieties
so I'll go back for another session
and hope it yields a good lesson

a dream

midnight and white roses
  open out like dove wings
   in the dark
little winds of thought
  rush through my ears and
whisper while the gentle rain
     falls
on the trees below our window

I am awake and asleep
  drifting through the deep
   dark and gentle rain
    while white feathers swirl
      and my thoughts unfurl

I will not remember this dream
  or what it can mean
but this I do know—
  I am drifting into a place of peace
with less trouble or worry or woe

early trip to new york

Drive to the station before dawn
    slow down so I don't hit a faun
Get to the station and park
    walk toward the tracks in the dark

suddenly the heavens part
    snow falls fast and hard
        passengers skitter
            and
        scatter
there's splatter
    and clatter

I look up and let the snow
    lick my face
        like a crazy cat

    and I tip my head back
    to taste the November surprise
of this icy sunrise

all aboard

Just across the aisle
staring straight ahead
no frown no smile
sits a woman
alone
my age or a bit older
folding and unfolding a piece of paper
she turns and I see her face
dead eyes
mouth clamped shut
staring
just staring at me
folding and unfolding
Is she thinking?
Is she awake?
Should I ask if she needs help?
I attempt a smile and she slowly
turns away
which makes me fear
one day I too may be on this train
just folding and unfolding . . .

the session

A walk to the shrink on this chilly fall day
makes me wonder what I'll say
when I reach the therapist
Something in the air
now makes me aware
I have little to share
so what do I say
when asked How Are You?
Are you happy or are you blue?
I'm a rainbow of emotional hues
and I'm looking for clues
to what I need to do
in order to feel in charge
of my endlessly large sense of
inadequacies
my lack of confidence
my fear of early death from dementia
and may I mention
I'm suddenly not feeling like talking
I'm kind of balking
at this session
and I don't want a lesson
on how to strategize
but now—
      surprise!
I'm at the doc's door
and before
I can turn and run a mile
she's standing in front of me
with a welcoming smile

cognitive behavioral therapy

"It's about exploring your relationships among your thoughts, your feelings
and your behaviors," she says.

And how does that work? I ask

"For example, when you say something to yourself like 'I can't do anything right, you can replace that thought with a positive expectation, such as, 'Most of the time I can do things quite well.'"

So just thinking something makes it so? I ask

"Practicing replacing negative thoughts with more realistic thoughts will help change thoughts that lead to low self-esteem into positive expectations."

OY, I think. That's a lot of replacing and I'm wanting to get up and replace myself someplace else . . .

"You reflect on how you can change the order of your thoughts," she goes on. "You learn to recognize the necessary steps that will help you think differently."

I AM SO OUT OF HERE! BUT I NEED A STRATEGY TO GET OUT OF HERE!

"You look confused," says she.

I'm not, I lie. I'm just thinking about strategies. That was something we started discussing last time and I think I'd like to talk about it.

"We *are* discussing strategies," she says. "Thinking differently is a strategy in and of itself."

In what way?

"For example—say you can't find your glasses and you look everywhere and you're angry at yourself and think you're hopelessly forgetful instead of thinking I need a strategy for not losing them. What might that be? Suppose I take a small bowl and put it in the front hall where I'll always leave my glasses when I take them off."

That wouldn't work for me, say I.

"Why?"

I'd just forget where the bowl is.

"But what if you told yourself, as you remove your glasses – put them in the bowl."

I'd probably be thinking of something else and just leave them wherever.

"Once you successfully put the glasses in the bowl you'll remind yourself to do that each time."

OK I'll try it! I blurt, just so she'll stop insisting and then I feel bad that I sound annoyed which makes me feel contrite.

"I think you're very tough on yourself," she says. "And that's probably a longtime habit."

I come by it honestly. I was always pushed to be better, to be perfect.

"By your parents?"

Yes. But mostly by me, myself.

"Ah," she sighs. "There you go. Your strategy to be perfect might have had the opposite effect. As an experiment, how about telling yourself, 'I'll remember to put my glasses in that bowl and if I don't, I'll remember the next time I misplace them . . .'"

Forgive me for saying so, but that sounds really simplistic.

"There's nothing wrong with simplicity. If you replace unhealthy thoughts with positive thoughts, your thoughts will become more realistic. Your brain activity will change. Positive thoughts can improve your brain function."

You have the right to remain silent, I tell myself. So shut your cake hole. Just nod. Which I do.

"So," she says, "think about it."

"I will," I say, forcing a smile. "I really will."

still here

My big sister the doctor calls to tell me she was alerted by
the senior living community where our mother is spending her
final days to say that Mom is not doing well, not eating much,
not drinking and not speaking except "in a language no one
understands."

Our mother is 103 and ½. She's been a pistol until a few years
ago. With the constitution of a Shetland pony she's weathered
illness and a stroke and defied expectations of death-any-minute
several times. She falls, but like the Energizer Bunny she bounces
back up without any broken bones. Yet this time, it sounds as if the
grim reaper is just around the corner.

So off we go—me and my husband—on a long drive, and
when we get there we find Mom sitting at a breakfast table, holding
a glass of orange juice, eyes closed. Prying the glass out of her hands
is not easy. She does not respond to her name. But there she is,
sitting up straight in a wheelchair, looking well. She is less wrinkled
than I am, with a smooth complexion and a head of lovely white
hair speckled with gray. Loudly calling her name many times, she
finally opens her eyes. She stares ahead and when I try to get her
attention, she turns but doesn't recognize me.

It's me Mommy, I say. It's me! Genie! Your second daughter.
She mumbles something in her own language—a mix of Yiddish
and nonsense—she looks at me and doesn't seem to know who I
am.

We attempt feeding her but she turns away, silently refusing, so
we move her out into a big empty room. My husband leaves us to
be alone together.

I kiss her claw-like hands, I caress her smooth cheeks, I talk to her.
I tell her how much I love her. I tell her she's been such a wonderful
mother. She gazes at me, but her eyes are vacant. She's there but it
seems there's no one home. Is her screen a total blank? Does she
have thoughts? Any cognition at all? She seems peaceful. I hope she
is. I pray she is.

Settling into silence she gazes off into space as I plunge into
memories of
Mom on the beach, dancing on the sand, leaping and prancing and
taking my hand
Mommy fingerpainting swirling blues and greens, making bright
yellow birds
Mom in the garden on her knees planting pansies and roses and
Mommy baking cookies singing "The goose is getting fat, it's time
to put a penny in the old man's hat"
and Mommy fixing lunch with peanut butter and toast
Mommy sewing skirts and dresses and taking up hems, letting
out waists and pressing to make sure her girls would sparkle like
gems and Mommy sketching, doodling, painting, shaping clay,
inventing worlds of form and color in her most singular way,
Mommy sleek in her black velvet frock
making a bun with her hair
dressing for a night out with Dad
who lights up like a chandelier
when she comes down the stairs...

Soon my big sister the doctor arrives and gets Mom to animate
somewhat. And since it's lunchtime we return her to the dining
room where she's suddenly happy to eat. A towel tucked into her
shirt, she slurps soup and takes a drink of water. She looks robust
and healthy as a Shetland pony.

It's not going to be anytime soon, my sister the doctor says
as she spoons sustenance into Mom's mouth. And we all nod.
Probably not today. Not tomorrow . . . but the winds have shifted,
and she's not long for this world.

I think she's got another year or more, says my husband

Could be, says my sister the doc. But probably not. And we
gently hug and kiss this woman who has lived so long, seen so
much, done so much. She's still here . . . but clearly headed for
another realm. Oddly I've always thought that since she's thirty
years older than I am, that means when she passes away I will live
30 years more. But at 73 I'm cloudy. At 73 she was skiing downhill
like a demon, painting, and making ceramic statues and having
absolutely no problem like forgetting words

or worrying about losing her mind

thanksgiving

It's
here
again!
The day of giving thanks and eating way too much and feeling like
a dirigible but enjoying family and friends and time off to walk
around in the
crisp fall air and discuss the disgusting state of affairs the world is in
and to tell jokes and watch movies and look at family photographs
and eat some more and drink good wine together and take a hike
to walk off the twelve pounds you've just put on and revile yourself
for doing so but what the hell when you go back inside there are
cookies and cake and just one more won't kill you and the kids
make you laugh and jokes abound and we stay up way too late and
then getting up in the morning is like rolling a boulder uphill and
the boulder is you and my husband announces that we should only
eat fruit today so he brings out a cherry pie
which makes me laugh and the sun is up and the sky is bright
indigo blue and my mind is for the moment clear as a bell and on
this day after Thanksgiving I am really and truly grateful to be
    A
      L
    I
     V
      E

as if by magic

Can't find it. Don't panic, I tell myself. Don't blame yourself, like the shrink said. Have a positive expectation. Relax. Start looking.

Go into the living room.

Not there.

OK.

Try the kitchen.

nothing!

Now upstairs in the bedroom. Where the hell would I have put it? Stop and think.

Breathe. It's just your wallet.

All your credit cards and 200 bucks!

It's not in my purse. But it's got to be in the house! I give up! But I can't! Then try something counter intuitive. Stop looking!

I flop into a chair, close my eyes and instead of beating myself up I think of nothing at all until suddenly I open my eyes and I remember where I left my wallet!

I put it in my flute bag so I wouldn't have to also schlepp my purse!

YES!

I think I may have discovered a strategy—when I misplace something—

I will not panic. I will look for it and if I can't find it

I will stop looking or even thinking about it

and soon . . . the answer will appear!

i consult with mrs. google

Feeling so proud of my strategic conclusion
I check with the seer to make sure it's not an illusion
and Mrs. G does not disappoint—
I learn within her depths that
deep breathing calms you down
and allows you to relax instead of to drown
in a panic of useless anxiety
opening your brain to regain
it's ability and agility
so you can vividly imagine what
you were doing or feeling
when what you've lost sends you reeling
NEXT:
"context reinstatement" can assist
in finding the memory you've missed
except I can't figure out
what the hell context reinstatement's all about
unless it's stupid simple, as in:
remember where you lost it—go find it
ELSEWHERE:
she offers a spiritual mantra
for retrieving things lost
from where they might have been tossed
which goes something like
Raajaa Baahu Gahatama Nasham Labyhate
and all I need to do is find a dedicated space
where I won't be disturbed
and chant that mantra
TWENTY-ONE TIMES

and what I've lost I shall be
    able to find

ANOTHER STRATEGY SHE SUGGESTS
      is simply to
    imagine whiteness!
      REALLY?
Instead . . . to keep a bit of politeness
    and not lose more of my head
      I think I'll just take a cold shower
                and go to bed

a dinner in new york

What is lovelier than a meal with a long time friend
    one with whom I used to spend
endless hours sharing joys and fears
    ups and downs
        loves and losses

while great food and wine seem to twine us together
    my words start to falter
    and my friend asks whether
I'm OK to which I say
    just tired and need to hit the hay

The check arrives and we both dive for it
    I win the war despite her protest
    but I lose the test
        in figuring out the tip as I slip
        the decimal point to the right
        which doesn't make sense
    then to the left but do
    I now need to double it?
        If only I had remained conscious during math
    I wouldn't be going
    down this slippery path
        It's getting too late to calculate
    so I approximate

Luckily my friend
                did not note my distress
      but
  I went to bed worried
                about my increasingly mental
                        MeSs

rescue animals

Early morning
on the farm
ALONE
husband at work
It's early winter
frost on the ground
and I'm trying
to write
to flute
but I'm feeling lonely and blue

I know what to do—
go outside to play with the dogs
two of them
who wiggle and waggle and jump and
make me laugh and
race after balls and growl and howl and want
more more more and we huddle and cuddle
and they may be animals who've been rescued
but today these creatures
are rescuing me

a lone wolf attack

early to rise
   with a sunshine surprise
wash my face
    then chase
 the cat
out from under the bed
  try to clear my head
turn on the radio
  only to hear
what we've all come to fear—
  a terrorist attack pledged to ISIS
in New York City and the crisis
was the work of one
with a pipe bomb and a gun

the explosion underground
 wounded three and it was found
  to be the work of "a lone wolf"
bound on a mission of bedlam
Is it now and forever us against them
 and can we find a way to stem
  the rising tide of mayhem?

to soothe with sound

In my life
when there's been strife
  and fear
or danger to those I hold dear
I free my mind
  by seeking to hear
    sounds that clear
the chaos I feel
  and more often than not
     it's the music of Bach
that restores my faith in humanity
  a reprieve from calamity
and offers
  a path
    toward
      banishing
     hopeless
      grief

I lie on the couch to listen and
  let the sounds of Bach
    wash over me like a gentle calming wave

at the intersection of hope and fear

Driving to dinner with my husband who has come back from a long day at work we talk about what we did and who we saw and where we went and I start telling him about having coffee with my friend . . . and I see the woman clearly in my head but my brain is holding her name for ransom, refusing to release it.

Oh God! She's my close friend, I groan. I just saw her!

What the hell is her NAME!!!!

My husband knows the task is to sit and wait until I figure it out. He knows not to guess. He knows to let it rest.

He knows by now that I like to retrieve the lost word or name by letting it sneak into my head like a cat burglar returning the stash.

Annette! I shout.

See! Says he. Just leave it alone and it comes back to you!

. . . except for the times it doesn't, I want to say
but I keep that
      to myself
because how long before my lovely man
tires of trying to help
    how long will it be before
retrieval
    causes
        upheaval

holiday visit with granddaughters
aged 3 and ½ and six

GRAMMY!!! they yell as they come hurtling through the doorway
bundled in down and bursting with energy. I pick each up, in turn,
and their delicious hugs and kisses make my knees buckle and my
heart turn somersaults.

    Can I sleep in the big bed?

                I want to! No, me!

        We're going to the circus! says one

        And to the museum! shouts the other. And you can
come!

    I reach over them to hug their mother, my daughter opus one.

      How was the trip? I ask her

    The usual—we started, we stopped

            one puked, the other pouted, but here we are!

    And in a New York minute we're off to the museum to show
the girls the dinosaurs the big blue whale and a film about the
universe and a trip to the playground where their mom used to go
and to Brooklyn for a sleepover with their auntie (daughter opus 2)
and the next day a trip to the Botanical Gardens and through it all
their laughter their energy their cuddles their endless delight

        leaves me breathless with joy

         and love and wonder

and even if all my words fail, I will always remember

        their delicious warm visit this freezing December

christmas morning in the country

SNOW   SNOW   SNOW
  lots of it
   buckets of it
    so sparkly bright
     the air so clear
    trees decked in white
    a glorious wintry sight

      Tromping across the field
      I look up at the blue canopy above
       surprised to be
      wonderfully worry free
        ergo
     on this gorgeous frosty day
    I will simply enjoy this silent
       silvery
       moment of
       PEACE

another frosted breakfast

Freezing again
   ice cold
      sub zero
waking up in the dark is one thing
   leaving the bed is another
but the dogs need food
    the cat demands attention
and coffee is to be brewed so that eyes can open

At the sink
   trying to think
moving in slow motion
I brew a potion
   while the pups go out
and come right back in
head to their beds and lick the
    lollypops of their iced toes

but my man has left us a roaring fire
   before leaving for work
and I and the beasts
    huddle at the hearth in the warmth of the flames

indolent me

I can't seem to do much today
    feeling numb
      and dumb
Could be the roaring fire
  but I desire
    little
which worries me
the once whirling dervish
who right now can't even finish
making the bed
or getting out the flute
to toot
or at least to try
which is why
  my fate
    may be to
take shovel   dig hole   crawl in
   close eyes and wait
     for a surprise
or better yet—hibernate

new year's eve party

we throw one each year
but it's clear,
        this was not a year many found dear
and politics aside

  I felt myself slide

    into fear and confusion

so

    I'd rather forget

two oh one seven

    it wasn't hell

    but it certainly wasn't heaven

And although there may be more loss than gain

        in what remains of my brain

I'm determined to reclaim

    whatever is left

in order to host our guests
and I will not stoop
   to be the party poop
      I will be ready to celebrate
        and to party
           hearty

frozen feet—warm hearts

The pups know what's up
as we prepare for the fête—
doing chores
    mopping floors
 moving chairs
    hanging lights
preparing delights
the hounds rush around
on the frozen ground
knowing what's up
while the cat strikes a pose
on her bed near the stove

At night it's zero degrees
and we worry that the freeze
will keep guests away
but friends come in droves
and we clink glasses make music
transpose a year that's been dreary
into one that ends on a   warm   joyful   note

as if by magic

Suddenly it appears
on the first night of the New Year—
the SUPER MOON!
238,900 miles from the planet earth
upon which we attempt to thrive
shining its brilliant light
and its perfect fullness
on the crisp white snow below

to look up
is to gawk to ooh to aah
wondering who switched it on
this megawatt bulb
this heavenly trick
is it a divine sign or
a threat to mankind

Meanwhile temperatures dive
penguins are at risk
sharks are dying
dogs are wearing boots—
Is the devil in cahoots with the sun?

and next—a bomb cyclone

It is predicted that
a sharp drop in atmospheric pressure
   will tonight slam the East Coast
      So are we toast
Or is it just another weather event
   we think we'll easily circumvent?
   but
what if the rotating winds truly converge
the waters surge
as the winds twist and twirl
and hurl debris and destruction
what then?
Let us pray
It will simply go away
and one day we'll be able to say
it was just a windy alarm
we got off without any harm
   but if
it's the apocalypse
   I'll pray for return tix
     as we are sucked up into the air

the big freeze continues

Even the dogs
   take pause
when escorted out
   to race about
They stop in their tracks
and turn their backs
 against the whirling snow
and rush back in
   to plop near the fire
having no more desire
   to be so bold
as to brave this kind of cold

Tomorrow promises worse
we pray the pipes won't burst
so just to stay warm
we huddle and cuddle
which is hardly a curse—
in fact it's a charm
offering pleasure
instead of alarm

my new years resolutions 2018

I resolve on this day
to hold anxiety at bay
to cancel fear
and keep my head clear
I'll let my mind
try to find
words
that aren't blurred
dates I can recall
tasks to do
both large and small
the right notes to play
things to properly say
I'll turn off the water in the sink
I'll go back to see the shrink
I'll remember which train to take
and when making steak—I'll broil not bake
I'll be courteous and alert
polite, not curt
and when I forget or fumble
I will try not to tumble
into a self-deprecating mumbo jumbo

the big melt

We wake to pummeling rain
which washes off the snow
but makes driving slow
last night it was minus seven
and this morning it's warming fast
by lunch it's in the fifties
and it's nifty
to walk outside without freezing
but the news leads us to believing
it will freeze tonight leaving us iced in again

By morning the prediction is another conviction
 the driveway's a skating rink
the car battery is dead
the cat won't leave her bed
the dogs are full of doubt
when doors open to let them out

Stuck inside we slide onto the couch
wishing for a kangaroo's pouch
so whatever can we do today?
duck and cover and listen to horses neigh

the shetland pony

If you want to come see Mom to say goodbye, it should be as soon as possible. That's what I was told and so on this cold and wind swept morning which happens to be Martin Luther King's birthday, we get in the car, my husband driving and the two dogs in the back seat—which is usually a treat for them until they realize it's going to be a very long drive which they will have to survive with biscuits and a few stops for stretching their combined eight feet . . .

Arriving at the rehab center where there is splendid and compassionate care we walk the long corridors to the nurses desk where we leave little cakes to thank them for their empathy and kindness
        and then we enter Mom's room
My sister the doctor is seated beside her. Mom is on her back, rubbing at her forehead. Legs twisting and body wriggling, she's struggling and seems to be in pain. A nurse comes to give her morphine and a sedative. We swab her lips with a small moist sponge and kiss her forehead and talk to her. My sister says it won't be long, maybe tonight, maybe tomorrow. Mom is definitely on the road to the hereafter which she here-to-fore has had a talent of evading but now the grim reaper seems to be in the room and is settling in for the duration.

I gently pull Mom's hands away from her forehead, and kiss her cheeks. Her eyes are closed her face is smooth and her melancholy beauty pierces my heart. I want her to go gently to sleep but I also want her to stay, I want her to wake up like the Energizer Bunny she's always been, but maybe at one-hundred-and-three-and-ten-months she's ready to slip away, to sleep. I want her to wake in a cloud next to her husband who has preceded her upstairs by 24 years. I imagine Mom primping for their reunion in the sky. She once announced, "I'm old and your Dad died young and I wonder when we meet up in the hereafter, will he find me attractive?"

Now before I leave her room, before I never see her again, I lean close and kiss her forehead and tell her how much I love her, how I will miss her and never forget her, and how I'm absolutely positively certain

that when she is united with her husband

he will find her more beautiful

more wonderful

more enchanting than ever

and I imagine the two of them

waltzing off into the billowing clouds

dancing gracefully together

cheek to cheek

dust to dust

They are gone, both of them—father, now mother
Gone. Vanished. What remains
are the memories I choose to keep
those that warm me when I sleep
the talks the walks the trips
the laughter the quips
the good times together
and the ups and downs we all weathered

A handsome pair, those two
with a zest for life and a deep love for each other
and for their 3 children
and 7 grandchildren and 12 great grands

now
I pray   they will peacefully abide
under the earth
in silence
side by side

days later—train to city

Going in
    things to do
        check for mail
            read letters open bills
                forage for food
                    then

I go to the funky drugstore on the corner which reminds me of my Grandpa's which was crammed with "sundries"—bottles of pills and jars of creams and scissors and brushes and soaps and plastic bath toys and dental floss and toothpastes and shelves of hair products and strange candies and I know I can get it all cheaper at CVS but this store is a memory bank, where I imagine Grandpa Morris who could play tunes on a comb and taught me a hand game called "Hock Pollak" which means Hit the Polish Guy and when it's my turn at the register I ask for my prescription and I am asked what it's for and I can't remember the name of the drug.

"I don't remember the name of anything!" says the saleswoman behind the counter. "It used to bother me. But now I don't give a damn. I might remember later on or the next day. Who cares?"

I laugh, having been caring way too much about my own memory or lack thereof.

"Here you go!" she says, handing me a small bag with my mystery meds which, when I exit the store, I realize I've left on the counter.

alone in my new york city apartment

The letters and magazines and bills to explore—
    all of which I decide to ignore
Except one email—from a high school friend whose sister has
died.
I reply with empathy and care and there on the e-address line are
a list of a group of friends with whom I haven't been in touch for
many years.
I stare at the names and I remember their faces and places where
they lived and
the things we did together and the parties we had and the close
dancing and holding hands and laughing and playing and applying
for college and hoping and praying
for our first choices and raising our voices to cheer Yay Rah Rah
Class of 62!
which was 56 years ago and I never went to a reunion I never
looked back
I forged ahead as we all did to become adults to have new lives new
friends
new adventures but now more than a half century has passed and
now that
there's more behind than ahead and now that both my parents are
dead
I find myself staring at the address line with emails of my high
school
friends and I feel an urge to reach out to them because they were in
my life for years and they knew my parents, they spent time in our
house, we were a group, I feel the need to make contact and so I sit
at the computer and write:
Hi to my Hall High Homies—

Since some of you may remember my mother, Shirley—I'm sending this to you—she lived an astonishing long life—103 years and 10 months!

(see screen shot below)

hoping to catch up with some of you at one of the next Hall High happenings.

Fondest wishes, Genie

i've got mail!

They wrote back—quickly—so many of them—with kind and
caring notes:
"I am flooded with memories of your home
    and how magical it seemed to me"
"I still laugh remembering your father driving us to school
    and telling us we should think about God as a lobster"
"Your parents were so smart and inspiring"
    "The picture of your Mom is great"
"Sleepovers at your home triggers warmest memories"
"Sending sincerest condolences"
"No matter how old losing our parents is so painful . . ."

Painful, yes, but the unexpected outpouring from old friends
with whom I haven't kept up fills me with love and remorse
and inspires me to connect with them now—now that none of us
have endless time left, now that there's more behind than ahead,
and ahead is a place that, for me, has an element of dread—
    Enough thinking about my empty head
    it's time to reach out instead
        to connect   not reject
to celebrate what's left and not be bereft
    make a new plan   do everything I can
        to carpe the old diem with gusto before my mind goes busto!

new treatments for you-know-what

I'm reading it, hearing it, seeing it—
clinical trials and new treatments for
    You-Know-What
the scourge that can't be conquered—
not yet—but maybe sooner than later:
This very day I heard on the news
evidence that a drug used for diabetics
may be effective for treating You-Know-What
It's theoretical at this point but FDA
approval is moving it along
in a priority review and
the drug may be repurposed
and ready soon
at an affordable price
which would be nice
I should be excited but I'm not delighted
the thought of being treated
makes me feel defeated—
I don't wish to admit that I need to take a pill
I'd rather heal my brain with sheer will
call me a jerk
but I bet it can work

get real

OK I admit I'm in denial
Should I sign up for a drug trial?

First I'll do research and see what I can find
that will quell my fears and clear my mind

A LITTLE HISTORY
I learn: in 1906 Dr. Alois Alzheimer first described "a peculiar
disease" and in autopsies he found dramatic shrinkage and
abnormal deposits in and around brain cells

The invention of the electron microscope in 1931 allowed further
study of the brain and the first validated measurement scale for
assessing cognitive and functional decline in older adults paved the
way to correlate the level of measured impairment with estimates of
the number of brain lesions and the amount of damaged tissue
    MY QUESTION: Were these older adults alive or dead when
tested?

    (that's a morbid little joke)

when i was 4 years old

In 1948 a unique cerebrovascular amyloid protein became the
prime suspect in

triggering nerve cell damage—beta-amyloid was identified as a
possible trigger of

nerve cell damage. Then, a "bullet" was added to the trigger—with
the finding of

the combined presence of two classes of abnormal structures . . .
amyloid peptides

and something called tau (sounds very zen!) can self propagate and
spread

through the brain and screw it up even more... so plaques
and tangles and cognitive impairments start messing with the
destructive biochemical pathways they initiate. . . .
          NOTE TO SELF—FACE IT—YOU'RE TOAST
BUT KEEP CALM—AFTER ALL THAT WAS THEN AND THIS IS NOW
                    AND NOW in 2018
     Every large drug maker is developing antibody treatments
to attack the amyloid protein (SEE ABOVE) that builds up plaques
in the brain
and there's something called phagocytosis which is a process in
which the
                brain cleanses itself
NOTE TO SELF—I imagine a tiny mouse with a broom sweeping
around inside my gray matter

(STAY FOCUSED)

In 2018 I read that there are hundreds of HOPEFUL studies:
like one that pinpointed a piece of DNA that was thought to
prevent the disease

        BUT guess what?   Turns out it doesn't

seriously now

There are new immunotherapies and new medications
    SUCH AS:
    the Alzheimer's cure diet
(but I can't find out what you're supposed to eat)
    and there also are
    hopeful dementia breakthroughs
    HOWEVER—99 PERCENT FAIL TO BE EFFECTIVE

There are experiments and investigations of vascular and
neurogenerative
diseases and pathologies and hope is on the horizon with future
drugs but
    they don't treat the underlying disease
and several studies I read say it will be another HUNDRED years
    before the dust will clear . . .
    SO HERE'S THE DEAL
There are currently no meaningful treatments
    no prevention
  no interventions, no modifying therapies
    and currently
    NO CURE
Disarmed with this knowledge
  I go upstairs
    turn out the light
    and pull
      the covers
        over my head

my antidote to fear

Today I will flute
   I will flaunt my flute
   I will flute my flaunting
I pick up my old friend made of gold
   which makes me feel bold
   and what will I play?
the piece I start with almost every day
   SYRINX
   by Claude Debussy
   His musical portrait of the myth of Pan and Syrinx
   for flute alone:

The lusty satyr Pan eagerly pursued the lovely wood nymph Syrinx
who spurned

him. Luckily in those days nymphs knew a neat way to deal with
sexual harassment

METAMORPHOSIS!

Syrinx ran to the river and as Pan was about to catch her, she
begged the gods to

change her shape and just as Pan grabbed her she turned into a
bunch of reeds.

Disappointed, Pan sighed and the sound of his breath across the
reeds was the

sound of the first flute.

the piece is merely 34 measures long and lasts about 4 minutes to
play
    which I do almost every day and have done since I was 10

    when I imagined myself then
as that nymph and in my mind's eye
I would enter the mystical forest and
envision myself racing toward the water
        then
           diving in
    and
being
    saved
I can calculate that for 63 years
  I've played Syrinx almost daily
    always differently
  always dreamily
  I've performed it by myself for myself
approximately twenty-two-thousand-nine-hundred-ninety-five
times
    and
       I
    never ever
     tire of it
    and never will
because it's not some
    goddess
   that will save me—
   IT'S THE MUSIC

sun valley

Are we crazy to go?
NO
It's my husband's birthday #77
and Idaho in winter is heaven
It's where two of his adult kids live and thrive
and other offspring will also arrive
we'll ski and snow shoe and hang glide
and there are horses and gondolas to ride
all cares and duties and worries tossed aside
BUT
We land in the Valley where the temperature is fifty degrees
while back in the East there's a deep freeze
what's left of snow is sparse and crusted
but none of the gang are at all disgusted—
The air is brisk, the sky's a perfect blue
what we decide to do
is to take it in our stride
run on treadmills like mad fools
Swim in the steamy hot outside pools
then hike up icy trails
come down to dinners where laughter prevails
and the sad state of the world pales . . .

my sun valley strategy

At first a mood of high anxiety
I worry that the extended family
will see I'm losing my grip
they'll hear me starting to slip
up on words that aren't even hard

I need a strategy
that will set me free
and quickly I realize no one will care—
this is a vacation and to be fair
we're all here to have fun and to share

So at our first dinner in town
I put my fork down
and listen to the sound
of a happy group sipping wine, slurping soup
laughing and clowning and having fun
And best of all—
I could join in and be one
of them—all I have to do
is to do it
which I did do
and happily too

self punishment is not the best strategy

Sun Valley was delightful but the
plane trips to get there and back were frightful
not to mention the time change which knocks one off balance
and there's a fatigue factor that lingers longer than it should
and my husband is upstate and I'm back in my little New York
apartment where I find my mind lacking luster
plus simply unpacking leaves me wishing to lie down and close
my eyes and I'm not depressed I'm simply wondering what to
do next should I pay the bills or take some pills or go out to
forage for food or practice the flute or call my kids or go pick
up the mail or dust the windowsills—such conundrums
invoke doldrums and Melancholy Me is not who I want to be
so now I better find a strategy—how about Shape Up!
What's with the lassitude and negative attitude?
Maybe try being gentler, try giving yourself a break—
Get back to your Sunny Sun Valley mood! Don't punish yourself!
Just go slow and you'll know
    what it is
        you need to know.

but the next day

What's that word?
It's so absurd—
It's a place where I need to go today
but I can't find my address book
no matter where I look
please don't let this be my nasty fate—
to forget appointments and what they're for—
and now it's getting dangerously late . . .

Just chill, if you will, say I to me—
sit still, that's the drill. . . .
    AND
as if by magic – there's a tingling in my head
  and suddenly I know!
I have an exam
for a mammogram
I even know where to go
I'll dress in a flash
and then dash
off to my appointment
feeling like a
    total
     BOOB

waiting to be told

I have a daughter who fought the big C
she never complained despite surgeries and pain
and with two little girls at home she made it plain:
"I will not die. I can't," she said. "I won't."
She didn't. She was brave. She was bold
     SO
after having to inhale and hold my breath
while my breasts were squashed
and pressed and after nervously waiting
in a room that's too cold
There's no greater relief to be told than:
     EVERYTHING IS FINE!

I feel instantly divine having stepped across the line
from terrified to terrific and to be more specific
    I feel grateful and lucky
 I think of my daughter who vowed to be brave
 and I realize now it's myself I need to save:
I will not fall apart and wallow in the rubble
   of cognitive troubles
I'll find a way to keep them at bay
 and one by one
   burst them like bubbles

does this subway know
where it's going or is it me?

Off to a concert uptown to hear a friend perform
Looking forward to it even though it's a dark and stormy night
and there's little time and no taxis in sight so
I rush to the entrance of the Circles of Hell
otherwise known as De Blasio's Inferno
I descend filthy stairs to stand on a crowded platform
and wait . . . and wait . . . and wait
and wonder which circle of Hades I find myself in:
is it Limbo or Lust or Gluttony maybe Greed—nope . . .it's ANGER
It's getting too crowded, dangerously crowded
and everyone is ANGRY and seriously overheated
and then . . . then . . . then FINALLY two trains arrive, local and/
or express
and of course the smart thing to do is jump onto the faster train
since I'm in a hurry and I don't even mind being jammed up against
a pole with some guy breathing down my neck except that
when the train trundles out of the station I realize
something incredibly interesting—This freaking express train goes
to Queens!
I panic! I'm screwed! I'll miss the concert! I'm a jerk! an idiot!
until: SELF PUNISHMENT IS NOT A GOOD STRATEGY
pops into mind and instead of berating my dumb ass I hop out at
the next stop, rush up the stairs out to the street and what do find?
a nice neat Yellow Cab
                    which I grab
            and PS—the concert was great!

how can this be spring if it's february

Sunshine
    everyone smiles
it's charming
    almost alarming
there's a breeze in the trees
    and it's balmy
      which does calm me
I walk down the street to find a treat
    something to eat
while I watch college kids in shorts and tee shirts
    and the skimpiest skirts
sashay on their way to class or to what-the-hell skipping class
    and going to hang in the park
which is the kind of lark
    that's more a spring thing
      and I join in
sitting on a bench I look up and let the sun
    cup my face in its warm embrace
and for a moment, a lovely little moment
    it's as if all's well in the world
    and although it's pretend and I know it will end
      in snow sleet and hail I will not fail
      to remember this heavenly reprieve

a visit with the grand girls

Now four and six years old
so bright, so beautiful so utterly enchanting
I'm delighted to have them to myself tonight

We flop together onto their parents' bed
but I have no idea how to turn on the huge TV
I'll do it Grammy says the six year old
and she grabs three different remotes and shows me:
Olympic skating begins and cuddled together
we ooh and aah and the little one asks
Are you always going to be our Mommy's Mommy?
   Yes, say I—
  Until you die, right?
   Shhhhh! says the six year old. I'm watching!
  And after, do we go visit you in a cemenary?
 Cemetery, corrects the elder. Of course we'll visit Grammy
    Thanks! I say
     imagining that after my demise
      I might get a fun surprise
    two little angels visiting so I won't be alone
   throwing sweet flowers on their mother's mother's tombstone

up country — the first of march

Where's that lion that should scare us with a mighty bellow?
he pranced in like a pussy, a very timid fellow
all he brought was a cluster of clouds and a bit of sun
but the prediction for tonight promises no fun—
rain, then heavy snow and high winds
that's how the tumult will begin

    I've just come upstate from the city
where it's been warm and very pretty
    but here in the wild, there's reason to worry—
falling trees flying leaves and animals that scurry
And my husband is stuck at the airport in DC
    so it's just the dogs, the cat, the horses and me

I've got a fire going
    so far nothing is blowing
my husband arrives and we have a quick bite
then hurry upstairs to prepare for the night
    fingers crossed that the forecast is wrong
      and the winds so far are not that strong
So we'll be cozy and calm as clams
    and hopefully that lion will turn into a lamb

the storm

No howling winds to startle us awake
the house remains stable and doesn't shake
It started at midnight
when we weren't quite ready
a steady and heavy
heaping of snow
that kept us alert
hoping no trees would fall
or horses fly away
but now halfway through the day
it's a roaring blizzard and on its way
to an apocalyptic ending
sending branches flying
and lights flickering
and we know villages nearby
have lost all power
so we might be next—

But wonder of wonders
we wake up on March the two
and the sky is a marvelous cerulean blue

ducking the destruction

Trees down
power outages all across the area
we were so lucky
and grateful to be safe

In our small town
people look after each other
and make sure
the livestock are standing
the pets are accounted for
the neighbors are intact
in fact
I'd venture to say
that in every way
this small town
has a big heart
that beats with kindness
and concern
and has helped me learn
the importance of
  kinship
    and
      community

music after a huge storm

The show goes on
in the newly renovated opera house in Hudson New York
    and I, the artistic director for this music series
    will introduce the concert called PROTEST
an evening of defiant, passionate and ironic songs that touch on
some of the hot-button issues in today's news sung by fabulous
young vocalists

Full house—huge expectations, time for me to get up there

An Arts Correspondent on CBS TV for years
I had no worries or fears
but that was before my brain started leaking
and now when I attempt public speaking
my heart beats too fast and I fear fumbling
or ending up mumbling
I'm embarrassed to need a crib sheet
when my memory was once so complete
but as I approach the stage I tell myself
it's about the music not me
and I say my say and sit down to listen
to young voices that glow and glisten
like sunshine after a raging storm

mid february

I'm back in Apple town
my moods are going up and down
I'd like to find out why
so I think maybe I should try
to go visit the shrink
even though I don't think
it's much of a help
I haven't gone for many weeks
so what's the point
of an appointment
. . . on the other hand maybe . . .

at the shrink

I come in from the street
and find myself alert and upbeat
her office is warm and neat
and when asked how things are
    I find myself
talking about my concerts
    my trip out West
my this and my that
how I'm feeling really good
as I certainly should, but . . .

But what? she prods
I don't know, sometimes . . . I'm just sad
    Tell me about it says she
I swallow hard and say the first thing I think of:
    My mother died
    I'm so sorry, she says
Thank you, but it seems long ago and it's only been a month or so
and I haven't thought much about it I mean she was almost one
hundred and four and I hadn't been able to visit her often but I did
see her a few days before her death and I knew it was time I feel
remorse and emptiness and sadness but not grief because her life
was long and eventful and I never had a really close relationship
with her and I feel as if I mourned her maybe not properly but I
don't know if there is a proper way so I guess I said goodbye but
now sitting here talking about her oddly I feel closer to her. And to
my father.
    Tell me about that

They were such a pair. I think of them together. I see them together.
And to be fair I joke about my new status as a 73 year old orphan
and it's funny but it's also not funny because Mom's death does
leave a hole in my life and in my heart. She and my Dad knew me
before I knew me so now having lost them both . . . it's just strange,
it's lonely . . .

*Losing a parent at any age turns your world upside down
rollercoaster emotions, joy and of anger, sadness—and you're right that
there's no correct way to mourn. Just feel what you feel.*

I feel like a bad daughter. I haven't wept enough. I haven't
missed my mother enough. I don't feel empty enough.

*You do feel deeply or you wouldn't have come to talk about your
Mom, even if you didn't intend to. You arrived today feeling quite
good about yourself, but you do have a tendency to self deprecate. The
good news is—you're functioning well and mostly feeling better. There's
nothing that can replace the woman who gave you life. You need time.
Give yourself some time. . . .*

Back in my apartment I find myself spending the evening
looking at old photos, Mom's letters, her paintings, her pottery, the
jewelry she gave to me, the clothing she left behind and one special
photo I've had framed on my wall for many years—my parents,
on a beach, so young, so in love, with so much ahead of them, and
they're smiling at each other with infinite hope for a long and happy
life ahead of them . . . which I do believe

they

each—alone and together

truly

achieved

a concert to celebrate lenny b

at the exquisite Hudson Opera House in
Upstate New York
I'm the Artistic Director of this group
I've invited a terrific troupe—
Three fabulous singers (one of whom is my diva daughter)
and a superb pianist
and . . . me playing a short piece
I'm, as always, nervous—will we have a good crowd
will it be an evening of which I'm proud?
But this concert isn't about me
It's about a genius called Lenny
as in Bernstein—celebrating the hundredth anniversary
of his birth
an homage to his power charm and charisma
and I remember his Young People's Concerts
I watched them on TV
sitting on my father's lap
Listening while the maestro tapped his baton
raised his arms and set in motion
the most marvelous sounds I'd ever heard
and now, some seventy years later
my gratitude to Daddy couldn't be greater
for introducing me to music so sublime
that has sustained me for such a very long time

april fools day in greenwich village

Early morning and the trees
out my window
are sprinkled with fairy dust
or is that snow
NO
It can't be
but yes that white stuff is sticking
and I throw on clothes and boots
take the elevator down
to find slush on the ground
like coconut sorbet
I'd like a lick but for sure it would make me sick
so I lean down to create a snow cone
and there I am alone on the street
not willing to retreat—
Maybe the heavens are fooling us April Fools—
mixing Passover with Easter
Let's call it EastOver—
a new holiday
        mixing matzoh balls with Easter eggs
            and dozens of funny yellow
                marshmallow bunnies

am i the april fool?

Making a list and checking it twice
want to find out if my brain is on ice
Can't seem to hold a thought for more than a second
Names elude me, much faster than I reckoned
so I try to visualize friends' faces
But images fade fast and I need to rest
or get up from my chair
and take a stroll, or go out for fresh air
But the sidewalks seem precarious
and the few folks out there look nefarious
so why don't I pick up my flute
and start to toot
Nope, it's not even a quarter to eight
my neighbors won't think it's great
to hear me pipe a tune
like a wacko loon
so is this my fate
under blankets without my mate
worrying about my mind
which I can't seem to find
or am I just the biggest fool
on April's second day?

note to self

I'm worried I'm going back to square one
    from whence I've come
meaning my initial confusion
    feels now more like a contusion—
I've got a shiner where my brain used to be
    it's become more and more troubling to me

But I don't want to go to the shrink
    I don't even want to think
I'll just take a walk and wander
    and see where my feet take me out yonder . . .

There's a chill in the air but I don't care. . . . I stroll to the park:
Sun's out–kids on bikes–couples holding hands–buds pushing
up through the dirt–dogs barking–saxophones squawking–old
people talking–chess games in progress–robins singing–card game
in motion–someone applying sun lotion–basketballs flying into
hoops–ice cream scoops in paper cups–and a toddler attempts to
run and topples over but no harm done he's up in a wink and tries
again–and I picture myself as a young mother playing with my two
little girls and how lucky I was to raise them and love them and to
be loved back and by my grand girls–and thinking about love–I've
given it and taken it I've chased it I've wasted it but that was then
and this is now and now I vow to revel in those I cherish and to stay
close and give them the most love I possibly can before I perish

the mystery of making music

To play a musical instrument is to merge an object into thought and emotion that effects both player and listener. Which is why holding my flute and blowing across the mouthpiece to send sounds out into the world is an attempt to reach - to connect - to touch - to communicate in an ineluctable way - but to what - to whom am I yearning to connect?

some days I'm able to sculpt the sound,
    to flute myself into a different realm
        to take flight
other days it's as if I don't even know how to hold the instrument
      where to put which fingers
  how to shape a phrase or find the center of the sound
and then I feel like a boxer
      trying to get back into the ring
        after a blow on the head

To listen to music is—for me—like entering another realm, a higher cerebral system where sound and meaning blend together, where received music washes through my head and body and soul without the burden of having to move my hands or mouth or to let just the right amount of air to be expelled from my lungs. And which do I prefer—the ease of listening or the effort of shaping phrases that float and soar? Effort or ease? Choose one.

No can do.

Ergo I assume I desire both—

The beauty of received sounds that inspire and the desire to create special sounds of my very own.

It's a conundrum
a puzzle
a challenge
a mystery and
a riddle
now that I've passed the middle
of my fluteful life
I don't want any more musical strife
yet I know full well
I'll get up in the morning, put the flute together
and pipe on until the piping's done

april 14 2018

She may be gone
but I will celebrate my mom on this her 104th birthday
I will walk down by the Hudson River
on this mild and sunny morning and remember
Shirley Cohen Rich
who was born on the lower east side
whose sisters and brothers called her Shandel
who spoke only Yiddish until she was taken in hand
by a lovely teacher who helped her understand
English and to speak it
and she spoke it
with a heavy accent
but a light heart
a teacher who played music
and read books to her and other gifted kids
after school just to help them, just to give, to bolster
to inspire
Her teacher was Eugenia Bach
Hence my first name
Eugenia
and as for Mr. Bach
how could Shandel have known
how much her daughter would love to play
the music of that magical mystical marvel of a man?

revelation

I've just read in the newspaper that having writer's block is an early
sign of
      YOU-KNOW-WHAT
      Well if you please
It would have been helpful if I'd have known this a few years ago
    when I was struggling to put pen to paper
      which then seemed to be heavy labor

Now I find I write mostly in rhyme
    I have no idea why . . .
But when I allow levity and brevity to enter my head
    it seems to be my way of
      expressing what I know and feel
        separating what's fake from what's real
  and perhaps this stream of words is
 a way to show myself
  I'm not going out of my mind
   I'm going into my mind
and mind you my brain
  seems to have gained
  a sense of freedom and fun
I'm no longer holding an invisible gun
    to my head to get pages done—
I've now got a hunch I've got a bunch
    of ideas on which I shall happily munch and crunch

changing my tune right now

I've been obsessed about my diminishing cognition
But I'm now determined to turn on the ignition
and drive my fears away. It's time to improve my condition
Instead of waiting for it to get worse- I'll chase away the curse
   There are suggestions galore
about how to explore
  ways to keep your mind as vibrant as before:
    do crossword puzzles
     take hot yoga classes
      learn to play a musical instrument
    (been there done that - still doing it)
manage your money so you can go to Tahiti (or gift it to your kids)
  take a cooking class
    learn another language
      draw a map from memory
    cross train for your brain
       and if you eat right and exercise and meditate
      you certainly will improve your fate
       It won't be too late
    the effort might make you depleted
     exhausted confused and defeated
BUT POWER ON! POWER THROUGH!! IT'S GOOD FOR YOU!!!!

figuring it out by myself

Please don't bother me.
I'm meditating . . .
which means I'm not
because my mind is not empty
I am thinking of other things
than meditating
like not meditating
because I want to be working on something else
    like writing or practicing the flute or emptying my head
which I find impossible at this moment and I dread
    sitting here like a pretzel against the wall
getting no peace of mind at all
    because my mind is in pieces
and yet I bet if I could just make space
    in my cranium I could pick up the pace
and finish this half hour of nothingness
    thereby clearing the air
and getting on with things
  except now
      for the life of me
               I can't remember
             what
                   in the world I was
                      intending to do . . .

presenting the players

Another concert and as I'm the Artistic Director
I must go onstage to introduce
a terrific group—all women—a brass quintet :
I've written some notes about this remarkable troupe
that seem easy to say—but when I try speaking off script
I get tripped up
I can't remember what I need to convey
I forget which player plays what and I feel like a dope
So I'll ask my husband to listen and help me cope

As I started to speak I stuttered   I felt my face glisten
I couldn't remember a thing I'd written
my man spoke up:
Read from your notes—no one will mind—no one will judge you
But I judge me I blurted, sounding like a dopey diva

At concert time a contrite me stepped out on the stage
I read from my notes to introduce the night
It felt just fine   it seemed perfectly all right
the quintet played with energy and glee
the concert was dazzling and as for me
I learned an important lesson—and here's my confession—
What I can no longer do with ease I will find ways to do my best
and with trying—maybe I can I make my best better

as if by magic

this wicked winter has been whisked away by a warm breeze
and a soft shower has inspired bulbs to flower
overnight

I stand outside
in the early morning light
to see daffodils on the hill
tulips peeking through the ground
purple lilac buds about to burst open
forsythia bushes exploding with bright yellow blossoms
like burning bushes in the desert

Delicate pink blossoms swing from long thin branches
of a weeping cherry tree
Does she weep to shed the misery
of a hard and troubling winter
or are those tears of joy that nature has given us
a transitory gift to treasure?
I stand beneath these winsome blossoms with
astonished pleasure

relevantly related word

Damn! I need that music!
   I need it ASAP
  and I'm not gifted with finding stuff on the net
    but I won't panic. Not yet . . .
I'm going to give him a call—that guy—from whatcha call it—
that music place I contact when I need a score—I can't remember
the name of the store—or his name—I have to tell him what I
need and he'll send it—express mail—to wherever I am—but he
can't send it if I can't remember his name which I'm now furiously
searching for on my iPhone—how will I find it—I'm in a mini
panic, ok a major panic—and I try googling music stores in NYC
but none of the names are familiar—and I'm surfing a wave of
worry not to mention self disgust—
    I decide to take a walk and stop thinking about what I can't
stop thinking about which is what a dope I am and how I'm losing
my mind faster than a hound loses a fox . . .

    At least it's a lovely spring day. I'm up in the country and I
wander and wonder at the explosion of colors and smells and I calm
myself down and walk and inhale and think about the flowers I'm
eager to plant and the tomatoes and the kale and somehow, a word
comes to mind which is not THE word I've been seeking and yet
it's there, peeking around the corner of my brain and I grab it—
LEARNING! But what does LEARNING have to do with the name
of the store? And then the store name pops into my frontal lobe—
EDUCATIONAL MUSIC! That's it!

Now—when I'm filled with anxiety
    I won't worry about losing words

I'll just let them go
I won't wrestle with my head
I'll relax and
imagine some word that's related
or one I haven't anticipated –
and instead of getting twisted into knots
I'll allow myself a moment of grace
and the right word will fill the empty space

Am I on to something? As if with a butterfly net
I might capture the mot juste
without even trying?

I don't know the answer
but if I let a peripheral word
land in my brain like a bird
perhaps it will make a nest
and tweet a word that suits what I want to say best

word catcher

Seems I'm doing well and feeling swell
so what makes me want to go tell
the therapist
what's been happening to me?

I feel a need to expound
on the little strategies I've found
that are helping me feel strong
instead of helpless stupid and wrong

I take an early train to New York
the doctor opens her door
and now seated face to face
she asks how I'm doing

I say my thoughts are brewing
I've found a way to
catch words that tend to flee
I let them go
and they come back to me
with a comparable word or
one that's virtually similar.
is this a clever trick
or is the idea idiotic?

In fact I think it's clever
says the shrink
it's a way to take anxiety out of the equation
which then frees your mind to find a word

that's comparable—
your mind is porous
it lets you dip into your own thesaurus
and will help you find a useful synonym

I leave her office feeling encouraged
and reinforced
a big boost to my mood
and a positive attitude

The strategy is mine
which makes me feel fine
I know it won't work all the time
but I'd rather be able to catch a word or two
instead of giving up and feeling blue

tornadic activity — internal and external

The sky above turns a dark muddy green
    lightning zigs and zags through the sky
        crackles and slams the ground
           with ear splitting sound

I'm stuck on a train
    slowly headed to our upstate home
and the conductor says trees have fallen across the tracks
    we can't move forward and we can't go back

    Lucky for me some friends give a call
        Where are you? they ask
          I tell them my pitiful little tale and
just by chance they're on the highway nearby.

Do you need us to pick you up? they ask
    No! I say. It would be a hideous task
Nothing is moving there's nowhere to go
        wind rain and lightning are putting on a show
          you're in danger already! I'm fine!
        Keep driving! just go!

  We're coming, ready or not! they say
    Be there in fifteen!
      Such dashing men saving a maiden in distress!

    With good pals
    who offer such kind deeds . . .

I feel
less scared—more prepared
almost heady—feeling ready

I've kept to myself these last lonely months
not wanting to burden anyone with my worries
I've concealed best I can that my brain is draining
but my attempt to be congenial is straining
I know it's time to exist in a happier key—
It's time to change my tune
from minor
TO MAJOR

the cat moves on

Lulu who we found five years ago dying in the manure spreader
    has moved in with one of our kids which is better
for her and for us. A feral cat, she is now a hip Brooklyn pet
    and we're told she's happy as a kitty

If I miss her funny tricks like chasing her tail
    I have little time to wail
        about it
        because
the daughter who rescues dogs in Idaho
    without missing a beat
will deliver to us another new treat
        AND
        She's arrived!
A German wire-haired pointer mix
    who joins our two jolly Griffons
        as they jump and show off their tricks

The three snort and sniff
        and dart around
rolling on the ground
    leaping in the air
chasing and racing
    and gracing us with barks and riffs
    So now we have
Sassy
    Izzy
  and
    LUCY

with whom I'm instantly in love
     with her waggling
         stump of a tail
her dreamy eyes, her soft white muzzle

The other two
       don't quite know what to do
 There were just two.
   Now they are three.
      Will they all get along?
        We'll have to see!

trouble in tahiti

Bedtime
    reading
He on his side of the bed
    Me on mine
I'm reading a book about our local towns
    and I find one name that makes me frown
        AMENIA
where is it?
  Not to panic, I tell my brain
close your eyes and let thoughts drift
    and surely you'll remember . . .

    But nothing comes to mind

What happened to my clever trick to
    catch words that tend to flee
let them go
       and they'll come back to me?

I give it a few more minutes but then I just have to know:
 "Sweetheart, where's Amenia?"
He glances at me in surprise. Our eyes lock. I see the worry in his
gaze and he answers—
"You go through Amenia to get to the train station. All the time."
Right! I say softly and I feel my face flush.
    I turn away and he does too
        because of course I know where Amenia is.
          Except I didn't.
          Not for

those several fraught minutes
    I had no idea.
        NONE
. . . and I saw the look of concern
 and worry in his eyes and Immediately
 I knew he knew I really didn't know and how scary
could that be because I imagine what flashed across his mind was:
  So this is how it begins.
        The caretaking,
            the endless helping my once independent wife

Now he, the love of my life
  closes his book and turns out the light
      pulls me close
        and gives me a gentle kiss goodnight

But sleep eludes me
      I imagine the downward slope
            and worry about how my love will cope
when I turn into a blithering dope

SYRINX

I take my flute out of its red velvet-lined leather case
    pick up the pieces and put them together
the headjoint—the body—the foot
    then line up the three parts just so and
place the mouthpiece under my bottom lip
    as I do every morning
I close my eyes and imagine her—
    the lovely nymph Syrinx
dashing across the woodland meadow
    I take a deep breath
and release a flow of air to see her in my mind's eye
    as she sprints to escape the Saytr's grasp
and I, fingers touching gold keys, lead the way
But after the rubato section as triplets dash toward trills that
    lead to a high held defiant b flat. . . .
    I have no idea what comes next
what octave what note which fingers go where
    and a terrible fear washes through me
    as I try to find my way through the bramble of
wrong notes and scrambled garbled sounds
    I'm lost totally lost and frightened because
I don't just play this piece, I feel it, I dance it in my head
and to forget one note fills me with a dark and ominous dread

an early morning walk on the rail trail

I leave two dogs at home
  and take Lucy, the new pup, to roam
   with me on this luscious new path
    that winds through flowering bushes
  towering trees and rough cavernous
rock formations

The dog is not used to a leash or a
  harness but she's game to go:
"Lucy HEEL!" I try but she's on to some scent
   and I'm getting pulled and stretched like taffy
attempting to hold her back is making me daffy

As the dog drags me along
  I think of the wrong
notes I played yesterday
  and wonder if I'll be able to play
Syrinx without a glitch today
     OR
will the nymph hide behind a stack of hay
  and politely say "No way!
No duet with you today!

I travel back in my mind
to see if I can find
  the time when I could play
with ease without the written music in front of me
  and the truth

                    is
            rarely if ever

Sometimes I think it's because at age four
    I rode my tricycle
        down a hill
        and slammed into a stone wall
            hitting my head
                blacking out and all

I was put to bed but no one said
        let's take her to the doc
Kids do slam into rocks
        she'll be fine

Or maybe my brain was bruised
    when I fell off a swing
        and I got a lump on the coco
Did it make my noggin go loco?
I've asked my big sister the Harvard Doctor
        if she remembers my childhood accidents and she said:
            I do. But old memories are often exaggerated
I think your fall from that swing
        wasn't really such a big thing

            I have to face it
    my musical memory has never worked well
            remembering notes
                for me is like being in a boat
            with a hole in the bottom
            and I've forgotten how to float

But as I walk through the woods today
    while the dog leads the way
  I do recall what a great pianist had to say
    when asked about playing "by heart"

"I'm able to play from memory," said he
    "but why do it
       when I actually know
               how to read
                 music"

father's day

On this day of extolling our patriarchs
    I think of my departed father—brilliant, successful, aloof and
wish he had seemed more pleased
      with me and my choices
instead of pointing to things like bad reviews and divorces

    What he liked most was when I could post
    some success—like a good performance, a fine review, a finished
book

    But today, the day to raise a toast
        to my father, I also remember well
the joy of
    our close talks
        the walks in the woods
the jokes he'd tell
  I believe he did love us kids
        but he absolutely adored his wife.
      Their love was intense and ardent.
They'd often act like kids, those two
    and as a young girl I liked to capture them with my pen
      which I did often and over and over again
And here's some verse I've found to prove that true:

eugenics   by eugenia

Father was a seal.
I mean he was lying on the bed
    In his white BVD's
clapping his bare feet together
    And saying
I'm a seal aren't I ?
So he was a seal
    since who am I to say
    Look you're not a seal
so I let him clap his big feet together

Mother was a German soldier.
I mean she was marching around
    in her nightie
    singing German Lieder
    and yelling
Floogen Gafleegle or something
    and stomping her feet
        dancing.
I am a cross between a seal and a soldier
    And watching
      I too
        laugh

levity, even with brevity, is a good thing

These days I am most of the time
    enjoying my life
and I thank my lucky stars I've gotten this far
    dealing with my death sentence
  which I don't mean in a morbid way
I just have to say that I'm glad I've been given a chance
    to glance at what's ahead . . .
        and what's not

I'll continue to look for ways to navigate my negatives
  and create strategies that help me when befuddled
  I'll embrace cognitive behavioral therapy
    when I think I'm having trouble
  I'll take out my flute and pipe away
    reading the music in front of me each day
I'll keep trying to write even if it's not quite
    as fluent as it used to be
    but making the effort makes me feel good
If I keep trying......it might keep me from dying
    too
      s o o n

smiles of this summer night

Tonight marks the longest day of the year
    and the start of summer
  in the Northern Hemisphere

One of the earth's poles is tilting toward the sun
    which means on this June 21 the gods will have fun
      with their magic powers

Owls will hoot the news, dogs will bark
    there may be bonfires, and songs and dancing
I certainly note the horses are prancing

The gloom of a cold wet spring is gone
    and we will now don next-to-nothing
to revel in the cool breeze and do what we please

The Peepers are peeping, the fire flies are flitting
    and I find it fitting
  to gaze up to the twinkling stars
and say a small prayer for the life I've led
    and the one I hope to
        keep   leading

july the fourth, 2018

And what is this holiday for?
  What exactly are we celebrating?
certainly not what we were originally commemorating
The US of A is splintered and spluttering
  every citizen is upset and muttering
    about the dreadful state of affairs
the bickering and dickering and doom and gloom
  is felt in almost every living room
But we've weathered dangers and disasters for 242 years
    so let's celebrate . . . minus our lingering fears

what to do?

Light the grill
   try not to spill
      don your summer whites
enjoy the sun and the fun and don't fight
    over politics and the right
        to sound off as one pleases
just wipe the ketchup from your chin
   and let the fireworks B
        E
          G
         I N

it's too damn hot

Everyone is saying it a lot
because this is a heatwave in early July
   that's so damn hot it curls your teeth
and makes you want to jump in a lake
     and stay there for a week
We have one small air conditioner
      plus a few little fans
  because up here
it never crossed the line
    between hot and horrible
but now that line has been doubly crossed
  and one's mood is tossed into the dumpster
as in Good Grief
  why is there no sign of relief?
    BUT
  too damn hot is not
the end of the world
   it's a small inconvenience
     and a reminder
that sticky clothes can be washed
    so what if your mood is squashed
      try to remember
       you'll wish for a day like this in December

back to the nymph

I did it
   on this morning, in this heat
I picked up my flute, sighed into it
     and Syrinx came back to life
        just like that
I didn't beg, I didn't plead
     I just followed her lead
and yes she made me stumble on a few notes
     but she allowed me to dote
on favorite phrases and to pause
     when I pleased

Should I summon her up tomorrow
     or just wait until she appears
Is she sending a signal
     that practice doesn't have to end in tears
and perfection isn't the real objective—
     the goal is to shape the sound
        let it abound
and wrap around in my head
     until my sighs mirror hers
        and we're two together
          becoming one

despite recent failures

It's on the front page
of today's big time journals :
"Early Tests Raise Alzheimer's Hopes Despite Recent Failures"
My eyebrows raise and I praise
the genius of science—
there's now a drug that reduces the amount of clumps
of a beta-amyloid protein
that builds up in the brain.
Zapping the beta-amyloid clumps might hasten a cure!
BUT—how can they be sure?
As I scan down the page I read that the "promise and peril of
Alzheimer's research has caused wild swings among the stocks of
drug companies."
What a surprise—there's much money to be lost or made!
not to mention there are doubts that tackling beta-amyloid clumps
will truly do the trick—or possibly make you really sick

While I praise these attempts to vanquish the disorder
I'll bet you a quarter
it won't be anytime soon
not 'til the cow jumps over the moon
and this old girl won't be around to refurbish her head
she'll be ten feet under instead
NOT TO SOUND MORBID OR ANYTHING . . .
But
I'm plenty frightened
I try making myself enlightened
It helps prepare me but also scares me
I try my best

to stand up to the test
of grace under pressure
    but each day I'm less sure
I can succeed at pretending
    I'm OK

I forget more than I can retain
    each step forward I gain
causes me two back
    I lack
all certainty
    and I don't mean to complain
I manage to make it seem
    I'm still on the beam
but how many more years
    do I have
And why do my fears
    often outweigh
        my good cheer?

I've tried the recommended activities
    that supposedly keep
    joggin' your noggin:
    brain training games—they seem inane
Crossword Puzzles—I've always hated them, never could do them
    video games—not for me
    I'd rather take a walk or jump in the pool
Or prance around the house like a happy fool
    I'm beginning to think
    it's either swim or sink
    I'm weary of acting
        like a victim

so I will now give myself a stern dictum—
   get off your duff
you've had enough
     of the woe is me
You've made a good decision
   to stop and envision
a new chapter in your life:
    living in one place
   with the man you adore
shove anxiety out the gate
   and be the mistress of your own fate

time to consolidate

Summer in the country is filled with flowers
    and hikes and bikes and music
The city summer also has its many charms
And I'm privileged to abide in both
    upstate and down
       YET
 now it's causing me strife
I'd like more time with my man
       BUT
does he want more time with his wife?

      OF COURSE!
says he. Come up and live with me
    fulltime, not part

      Sweets! I say
    I love you with all my heart!

Yet . . . am I really sure I want to live up here on a permanent basis?
    Will I miss my little oasis in the Apple?
Change is scary . . . can I grapple with what's ahead?
      YES!
   To be partnered with such a loving man
     makes me believe I truly can

it's been more than a year

Since
    my first visit to the
        DEPARTMENT OF NEUROLOGY
    at the famous College of Physicians and Surgeons
way uptown
    in New York City

I've had a second visit some months back
      (which was suggested)
        I passed muster
and they won't make me take another cluster
      of scary tests—at least not yet

So I'm getting ready to pack up
    and move from South to North
   from the Apple up to Dairy Country
      to live full time with the man of my dreams
who seems happy with the plan
    and I'm hoping that I can
adjust and be robust and get things done
  planning concerts, making music,
romping with the hounds and enjoying the surrounds

a promise to myself

I vow to hold tight to the belief
that I can train my brain to work better again
  maybe not at its tip top
    but well enough so I can keep driving my car—
      I still know when to go
        and
      when to stop
I've got strategies for finding objects I lose
    like glasses and jackets and shoes
   and ways to let words return to my head
without crying and taking to my bed
   but I have bigger concerns
   that burn into my mind
     such as:
THE TRUTH ABOUT MY CONDITION
   from now on is it only about attrition?
    Losing words
inability to read
   forgetting where I'm domiciled
  burning down the house
    drowning in the tub
    tumbling down the stairs
   and other fears
       that won't be stilled—or killed or willed out of my head

and suddenly i'm weepy

I'm worried—about nothing and everything
    My husband leaves for work at dawn
giving me time to get up and enjoy the pups
    read the paper and drink two cups
of coffee before taking on the jobs of the day
        which are to
    pick up the flute and play away
      answer the endless emails
        make phone calls and take the meetings that
      need attending

there's nothing really wrong
      yet I'm suddenly not feeling strong
        about my move up to the woods
although I love the birds
    the flowers
        the morning light

  what I won't find a delight
will be tackling the packing
but that's a spoiled girl's remark
   and I know moving is never a lark
   so I won't sit here in the dark
I'll learn to shed what I don't need instead

much to do about packing

Books books books
  whatever will I do with all my books?
Abandon them after all these years?
  It raises my fears
that without them I'll forget these friends
  I've carted from home to home
      like
Colette who taught me about sex and love
  Jay Gatsby—his hunger for money, his love for Daisy
Scarlett O'Hara—selfish and uptight 'til she saw the light
  Jane Eyre the orphan with guts galore
Nathan Zuckerman—neurotic and funny as hell
    WELL
they'll all have to sit on someone else's shelf
      because
I'm downsizing
  I'm offloading
    I'm letting go
      of what is not needed
      of what preceeded
I will give away what I've hoarded
  in my closets, drawers and on my shelves
I'll lighten my load, I'll purge with an urge
and I'll surge upstate feeling that less is so much more

music music music

I have so much so many such a plenty
of scores and proofs and editions
manuscripts frayed and fondled
where will I ever keep it all?
If only I were good with digital tricks
I could easily fix my problem
with an electronic music stand
and a touch screen hands free
device which would be nice
but I have enough anxiety as it is
and just the thought of turning a page with my foot
while blowing across the flute
makes my apprehension acute
so I seem to be stuck
and out of luck
But hey, I'm seventy-three
   and in principle I'd rather save a tree
and
    go
       hands
          free
But I'm afraid
    it's not to be

yet more news about an alzheimer's cure

More info
   more optimism
      in multiple newspapers
     about that possible cure
but before we can be sure
        or even believe it's going to endure
there's caution suggested about
     undue optimism
raising questions from some
        about a positive outcome
   more extensive trials will be needed
   to know if the new drug
is truly effective
    SO
I choose to be reflective
   yet hopeful the corrective
will emerge
  and there will be a surge
of hopeful happy seniors
    no longer scared
   and their sagging brains
       will begin to repair!

it is not fun but it's getting done

The boxes
    the packing
the piles of books and papers
  endless bending and hauling
    it's completely appalling
but friends, kids, and husband help
  and I start to enjoy the
    ferretting out
of what I want to throw away
  and when I divest
    it feels better than best
    and I've got to say
there comes a moment of delight
  when the movers
appear
  with their gear
and take the stuff out the door
The only problem will be at the other end of the move
  when it will behoove me
  to put things in order
But not to despair—
  I'll sniff the clean country air
    and feel lucky to be up there

a super sunny sunday

Almost August
   and the tomatoes are bulging
on their vines
   the flowers continue
to burst toward the sky
   in colors that astound
while on the ground
   our once hearty kale
   has been ripped out by rabbits
who attack at dawn
   and are gone
     in a flash
leaving the crop tattered and torn

   Nothing lasts forever
not kale or tomatoes or cucumbers
   or the glorious flowers that fill our fields
    or the people we adore
     and though I know my days are numbered
    I feel unencumbered
     by thoughts of my demise

    I do not embrace
   my inevitable decline
    but I'm determined
     to find
a way to make the rest of my stay
   on this problematic planet

filled with light
　　and love
　and
　　　music
As for the deer suit I promised to don
　I don't think I'll put it on
not now　　not yet
　I'm not ready
　　　I feel steady
　and I have a strategy to keep on keeping on
　　　which is simple:
　wake up
　　fetch the flute
　　　　summon up Syrinx
　give thanks for another day
　　and then
　play on!
　　　play on!
　　　　play on!

EUGENIA ZUKERMAN is an internationally renowned flutist and writer. She was the artistic director of the Bravo! Vail Valley Music Festival in Colorado for 13 years and the arts correspondent on CBS *Sunday Morning* for more than 25 years. She is the author of two novels, two works of nonfiction, and numerous screenplays, articles, and book reviews. Born in Cambridge, Massachusetts, in 1944, she graduated from the Juilliard School of Music and lived in New York City for many years. A mother of two daughters and two grandchildren, she makes her home in upstate New York with her husband, two horses, three dogs, and assorted wildlife.